The Art of Roughhousing

Good Old-Fashioned Horseplay and Why Every Kid Needs It

By Anthony T. DeBenedet, M.D.
and Lawrence J. Cohen, Ph.D.

Illustrations by Carl Wiens

QUIRK BOOKS
PHILADELPHIA

Copyright © 2010 by Anthony T. DeBenedet, M.D., and Lawrence J. Cohen, Ph.D.

Library of Congress Cataloging in Publication Number: 2010941012

ISBN: 978-1-59474-487-7

Printed in China
Typeset in Rockwell, Sabon, and Trade Gothic

Designed by Doogie Horner
Illustrations by Carl Wiens
Production management by John J. McGurk

Quirk Books
215 Church Street
Philadelphia, PA 19106
www.quirkbooks.com

10 9 8 7 6 5 4 3 2 1

*To my wife, Anna—a champion of play
and the heart of our family*

*To our children, Ava, Mia, and Lola,
who constantly bring immeasurable joy
into our lives*

*And to my parents, Karen and Nelson,
who have supported me every step of
the way*

—Anthony

*To my wife, Liz, and our children—my
wrestling coaches—Emma and Jake*

*To my parents, Ruth and Alvin. They may
not have roughhoused, but they never
stopped expressing love, affection, and encouragement in every other way*

—Larry

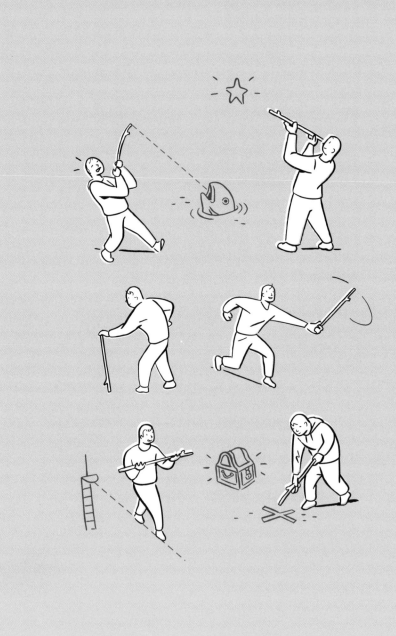

Table of Contents

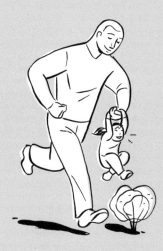

A Note of Caution

Roughhousing is great fun. It's also a little dangerous. In fact, roughhousing is great fun *because* it's a little dangerous.

And if you roughhouse with your children often—as we do—you should expect that someone will eventually get hurt.

Here's the thing: We believe that occasional bruises and scrapes are a normal part of childhood. It's how we learned to pick ourselves up, dust ourselves off, and stay in the game. It's how we grew our confidence and discovered the laws of physics.

We're counting on you—the responsible adult—to monitor your child and keep these bruises and scrapes to a minimum. We want you to have fun. We want you to get rowdy. But we need you to use common sense. If your child seems too young to ride a mattress down a staircase (page 152), give her some time to grow. If you have trouble lifting a suitcase into an airplane overhead compartment, please don't attempt anything like the Balloonist (page 56).

The publisher and authors do not claim that the information contained herein is complete or accurate for your specific situation. The publisher and authors do not endorse or encourage any irresponsible behavior, and specifically disclaim responsibility for any liability, loss, damage, or injury allegedly arising from any suggestion, information, or instruction in this book. We urge you to obey the law and the dictates of common sense at all times.

End of cautionary note. Now get ready to rumble!

Anthony's Preface

Growing up, my dad and I always interacted in a physical way. Although a regular old hug was rare, the exchange of arm punches, high fives, and bear hugs was commonplace. I think this type of affection was most natural for my dad. To this day, we still occasionally greet each other with a friendly slug or two.

Fast forward to 2007: Now I'm the dad. My friend David Fuelling and his family came to visit my family for the weekend. At some point, he and I were roughhousing with our kids on a rug in my house. As we rolled (and ran and flew and jumped) around, I wondered if anyone had compiled a book of rough-and-tumble activities for parents to enjoy with their children. The next day, I searched for the book online and found nothing. Soon I was delving into scientific research on play, which confirmed what I already intuitively knew: Roughhousing offers kids tons of physical and psychological benefits.

As I learned more and more about the science of roughhousing, I realized I needed to recruit an expert to help me write the definitive book on the subject. In my research I had stumbled upon *Playful Parenting*, written by Lawrence J. Cohen, Ph.D., a Boston-based psychologist who specializes in play therapy. Larry's book had a chapter on roughhousing that I particularly liked, so I set up a phone conversation and he quickly agreed to jump on board as coauthor.

If you're looking for something to turn your parenting world upside down (literally), then this is your book. As my mom always says, there are no do-overs in parenting. So let's play!

Larry's Preface

Unlike Anthony, I am a recent convert to roughhousing. My dad was not a wrestler, and neither were my three sisters. For me, as a kid, "wrestling" meant getting the crud beaten out of me by bigger, stronger, and meaner boys. So I avoided it when my daughter Emma was little. But parental love is a powerful force. I can't imagine anything besides my love for my daughter that would have compelled me to roughhouse with her. When I saw how much fun Emma had when she wrestled with other people, I forced myself to dive in.

Soon I was a zealous believer in rough-and-tumble play, and I started spreading the word. And then . . . nothing stays settled and easy when you're a parent, does it? Around the time Emma became a teenager and we cut back on our wild roughhousing play (but never cut it out entirely), I suddenly had a whole new wrestling challenge. Along came my 10-year-old step-son, Jake, and I had to learn a new set of rules, which basically revolved around *me* not getting hurt. Jake wanted to go all-out, and we bonded over our screams (some real and some fake) that drove his mother out of the room in a panic.

So if you have any hesitations about roughhousing, I give you a special welcome to this book. If you don't, I invite you to read on and take it up a notch!

CHAPTER 1

Our Bold Claim for Roughhousing

"It is difficult to capture . . . real-life play in words. But the overall impression given by practically all mammals is a flurry of dynamic, carefree rambunctiousness."

—Jaak Panksepp, Ph.D., in *Affective Neuroscience*

You know roughhousing when you see it: wrestling, pillow fights, jumping off beds, sliding down stairs. In this book, we give you a lot of roughhousing activities, but first we'd like to explore the philosophy behind all the horseplay. What is roughhousing all about, and what does it mean for you and your children?

Roughhousing is *play* that flows with spontaneity, improvisation, and joy. It is free from worries about how we look or how much time is passing. It is *physical*, and it promotes physical fitness, release of tension, and well-being. Roughhousing is *interactive*, so it builds close connections between children and parents, especially as we get down on the floor and join them in their world of exuberance and imagination. Most important, roughhousing is *rowdy*, but not dangerous. With safety in mind, rough-housing releases the creative life force within each person, pushing us out of our inhibitions and inflexibilities.

Rowdy, physical, interactive play is by far the most common type of play in the animal kingdom. It occurs in every species of mammal and in many nonmammalian species as well. We've all seen videos of lion cubs wrestling, but you'd be amazed by the vast number of species that enjoy rowdy play—elephants, whales, even ants.

The first person to explore the science of roughhousing was Harry Harlow, who observed young rhesus monkeys in his animal psychology lab at the University of Wisconsin during the 1950s and '60s. Harlow noticed that the monkeys often practiced what he described as "rough-and-tumble play." He was working during a time when many scientists did not consider play to be a viable subject for serious research, but Harlow went ahead and documented this play-fighting in great detail. He observed that the monkeys often displayed a so-called play face—an open-mouth, teeth-bared expression—which looks fierce to humans but to other monkeys actually says, "Let's play."

Since Harlow, observers of human behavior have discovered that we are remarkably similar to rhesus monkeys when engaging in rough-and-tumble play. Human children have their own play face, accompanied by smiles and laughter, to signal that roughhousing is play and not aggression. And, just like monkeys, roughhousing children will run, chase, jump, flee, wrestle, fall over, and play-fight. Playful hitting uses an open hand (as opposed to a fist) and much less force. The roles of the aggressor and the victim are fluid. In rough-and-tumble play, children—like young monkeys—will take turns being the chaser and the one being chased, the pinner and the one being pinned.

The State of the Art

Sadly, among many of today's families, roughhousing barely limps along on life support. What was once a motto of Safety First has evolved into a fretful new motto of Safety Only. Many parents are more frightened by skinned knees and bruised feelings than life's real dangers: stifled creativity and listless apathy. Some schools in the United States are even being built without playgrounds.

We've met parents who worry that roughhousing gives kids Attention Deficit Hyperactivity Disorder (ADHD). Not so! They fear that roughhousing makes kids wild, aggressive, and impulsive—and always escalates into chaos and anarchy. The result is that many fathers, with a natural instinct for rough-and-tumble play, are sidelining themselves; they read books to their children but don't dare to wrestle with them. New technology is partly to blame, too. Kids spend much more time in front of screens than they do outside.

And when children aren't staring at computers or TVs, they're being overscheduled, overprotected, and underadventured. Children's "playtime" is now dominated by adult-organized, adult-refereed, and adult-structured activities. Certainly, adults do need to be vigilant against abuse toward children, but that doesn't mean that free-form, rowdy play should be off-limits. Otherwise, children aren't really playing—rather, they're *being played*, by us, on our grown-up game board.

That's the sad state of roughhousing, in a nutshell. Yet hardcore roughhousers like us are always up for a challenge. What could be more exciting than setting the record straight and giving our art a shot of adrenaline?

The Bold Claim

Play—especially active physical play, like roughhousing—makes kids smart, emotionally intelligent, lovable and likable, ethical, physically fit, and joyful.

We're not exaggerating (much). Roughhousing activates many different parts of the body and the brain, from the amygdalae, which process emotions, and the cerebellum, which handles complex motor skills, to the prefrontal cortex, which makes high-level judgments. The result is that every roughhousing playtime is beneficial for body and brain as well as for the loftiest levels of the human spirit: honor, integrity, morality, kindness, and cooperation.

Roughhousing Makes Kids Smart

Animal behaviorists have observed that the smarter the species, the more its youngsters engage in physical play. Roughhousing releases a chemical called brain-derived neurotrophic factor (BDNF). As Margot Sunderland writes in *The Science of Parenting*, BDNF is like fertilizer for our brains. It helps stimulate neuron growth within the cortex and hippocampus, both of which are vital to higher learning, memory, and advanced behavior such as language and logic. Put simply, play makes animals smarter.

When a child and parent roughhouse, they activate various areas in each of their brains, including the pathways for motor coordination, creativity, and emotional attachment. This coordinated activation builds brain-cell connections, which is another way to say that it builds intelligence.

Such an association between play and intelligence makes perfect sense. One way to gauge intelligence is to observe how a person reacts in new and unfamiliar situations. The world is a complicated place; you can't memorize a list of correct answers to help you navigate every possible encounter. As Marc Bekoff and Jessica Pierce note in their book *Wild Justice: The Moral Lives of Animals*, physical play trains mammals to cope with the unpredictable; it makes their brains more behaviorally flexible and increases their learning capacities. That's true for ants, for polar bears, and most especially for kids—who can learn complicated concepts, like trust, by roughhousing with Mom or Dad.

When we say that roughhousing makes kids smart, we're talking about building foundations for academic success. Roughhousing boosts school performance. The fun of parent–child physical play may be what helps children learn language so fluently. Our playground hero, Anthony Pellegrini (a professor of psychology at the University of Minnesota), has reported that children's behavior on the playground—including how well and how much they engage in roughhousing—predicts their first-grade achievement better than kindergarten test scores do. More generally, Pellegrini finds that free play, especially when it includes the freedom to engage in roughhousing, improves everything from test scores to peer relationships in school.

This information raises an obvious question: If roughhousing is so good for academic achievement, then why are an increasing number of U.S. school administrators banning physical contact? In March 2009, a Connecticut middle-school principal instituted a "no touching" policy in response to an incident between two students. In a letter to parents, the principal wrote: "Observed behaviors of concern recently exhibited include kicking others in the groin area, grabbing and touching of others in personal areas, hugging, and horseplay. Physical contact is prohibited to keep all students safe in the learning environment." We suspect these administrators are motivated by a misguided understanding of safety. No one can argue that violence in schools is acceptable. But under these new policies, even high fives and hugs are off-limits.

In his book *Affective Neuroscience*, neuroscientist Jaak Panksepp draws a close connection between physical play and learning. "During play," he writes, "animals are especially prone to behave in flexible and creative ways." He recommends that schools use rough-and-tumble play as a reward for, or even as a warm-up to, learning. Children might focus more if offered the chance to roughhouse, much as rats will learn a maze just for the chance to wrestle with other rats. Panksepp also suggests a novel program to prevent and treat ADHD: lots and lots of rough-and-tumble play. Not just to let off steam, but to rewire the neural networks in charge of attention span, motivation, persistence, and reasoning.

Another reason roughhousing is so good for learning is that it provides an opportunity for making mistakes without fear of punishment. Everyone learns better that way. Bekoff and Pierce have observed that, across species, transgressions and mistakes are forgiven—and apologies accepted—during play, especially when one player is a youngster and the other is an adult. If a wolf cub nips his mother too hard during a friendly wrestle, she will reprimand him gently but keep playing. That's probably the reason for the play face that Harry Harlow observed: During play, animals and humans need to constantly communicate the message, "Don't get upset with me if I mess up; this is still play." In good roughhousing, parents *respond* to rule-breaking or excess aggression, but they do not *penalize* it.

That is not to say that roughhousing will make your child a genius. But as one factor that helps stimulate a child's intellectual development, it cannot be discounted. We may not have any information about Einstein's roughhousing history, but we do know something about the Dalai Lama's playful past. He relates in his autobiography that when he first began studying at the monastery, he had to be separated from his brother because they roughhoused so much!

Roughhousing Builds Emotional Intelligence

Being smart is about more than good grades and high test scores. To succeed in life, you need *emotional intelligence* as well. Play, especially roughhousing, promotes emotional intelligence. So when anxious parents ask us how they can assure their toddlers' acceptance to a good college, our answer is, "More play!"

Emotional intelligence is all about managing our own emotions and accurately reading the emotions of others. It's easy to see why these skills are so vital to success in adult life. It's also easy to see that young children are notoriously lacking in these skills. Roughhousing aids their development. In good roughhousing, you and your child practice revving up and calming down, which helps your child learn how to manage strong emotions. Roughhousing uses nonverbal communication to teach about emotions, which is much more effective than lectures. In good-quality rough-housing, you and your child also share lots of eye contact, and that's the best way to build up a strong ability to read—and care about—what other people feel.

Sometimes children will use roughhousing to showcase difficult feelings that are hidden under the surface. They may suddenly burst into tears, get angry, or even bite just when you thought the roughhousing was going great. Ava, Anthony's daughter, went through a biting stage at age two. It seemed as though every time they wrestled, she would, with no warning, chomp into Anthony's leg. After attempts at scolding (which didn't help much), Anthony stepped back to consider what might be going on. He realized that Ava usually bit him when he dominated the wrestling too much and didn't give her a playful and nonviolent way to conquer him in battle. Anthony also realized that the angriest bites happened when he came home from work later than expected. It was as if Ava tried to play once her dad finally came home, but suddenly she would remember her disappointment, and then out came the teeth.

Armed with this knowledge, Anthony brought these feelings into the open. He shifted his focus toward having more fun together. If he came home late, he would say, "Anyone who is mad at Daddy for coming home late, get in line!" Ava would giggle and get ready to leap on him. He always had a dishcloth or towel handy, so that he could hand it to Ava if she got the urge to bite something. Instead of trying to eliminate the biting through punishment (which probably wouldn't work and would have ruined the fun parts of the roughhousing), they figured out a way to accept those deep underlying feelings without having them come out in aggressive (and painful!) ways.

When we stay calm and welcome our children's feelings, we give them a safe and loving container for their emotions. Doing so helps children tremendously in the management of emotions that feel out of control. Simply sitting and listening to upset children is the best thing we can do for them; it allows them to get a handle on themselves. The success they experience in regaining self-control gives them more and more confidence in their emotional lives.

Roughhousing Makes Kids More Likable

It's common for parents to worry that their children will have difficulty making friends. Roughhousing can help. Kids who roughhouse are almost always more physically and socially adept than those who don't.

The connection between roughhousing and social success can again be seen in the example of Harlow's rhesus monkeys. Their play-fighting looks aggressive to us, but Harlow discovered that such activity was necessary for healthy social development. In fact, if young rhesus monkeys don't wrestle with peers, they're unable to mate when they mature. As the song says, "Birds do it, bees do it," but monkeys won't know how to do it if, growing up, they don't roughhouse with their chums.

One reason that roughhousing helps with being liked, and eventually with being loved by a partner, is that friendships and other relationships require care and maintenance. Boys, in particular, aren't prone to telling their friends, "I love you," or even, "I like you." Fortunately, they have other ways of showing affection. According to play researchers Tom Reed and Mac Brown, "Rough-and-tumble play provides opportunity for the declaration of friendship and caring relations." Today's preschool teachers frequently admonish boys to "Use your words!" but their natural instinct is to express affection with physical contact and play. Yes, it sometimes goes too far. But, more often, boys know just how far to take it.

Pellegrini found that well-liked kids engage in good rough-and-tumble play, whereas children rejected by their peers are more likely to engage in aggression. Upon interviewing students, he found that the ones who were well liked could easily distinguish play from aggression, but disliked kids had trouble telling the difference. The result is predictable: If you play-fight with someone who can't tell you're playing, you're likely to get a real punch back. Pellegrini concluded that rough-and-tumble play serves an important role in helping children develop social and problem-solving skills.

To be well liked, children need to be good at taking turns and at seeing things through the eyes of another child. In *Wild Justice*, the authors describe how animals will take turns when roughhousing. One will be the chaser and the other will be chased, and then they switch roles. Adults and their offspring reverse roles as well. Adult wolves will expose their bellies and necks to their cubs during play, something they would never do in a real fight, according to Bekoff and Pierce.

Panksepp describes a similar behavior in rats: "Play dominance clearly emerges if two rats are allowed to play together repeatedly. After several play episodes, one rat typically tends to become the 'winner,' in that it ends up on top more often during [wrestling] pins. On the average, the split is that the winner ends up on top about 70 percent of the time, while the 'loser' achieves less success, but the continuation of play appears to require reciprocity and the stronger partner's willingness to handicap himself." In other words, if the stronger animal insists on winning all the time, the weaker one will quit playing.

One of the secrets of leadership and negotiation is the concept of win-win: Everyone needs to walk away happy. Roughhousing is great for developing an understanding of this concept. If you rely on brute strength, you might end up with terrified followers, but you won't have any friends. Bekoff and Pierce note that, among animals, "Play only occurs if, for the time they are playing, individuals have no other agenda but to play. They put aside or neutralize any inequalities in physical size and social rank." Play will stop if one animal becomes too aggressive and only resumes if everyone communicates their readiness to be back in play mode. The pleasure of playing helps animals (and people) give up the power of force and rely instead on the power of friendship.

Roughhousing Makes Children Ethical and Moral

Bekoff and Pierce also claim that humans do not have a monopoly on ethics and morality. Many animal species share, cooperate, empathize, trust, act reciprocally, and agree on social norms. Guess what? The animals with the highest level of moral development also engage in the most play, especially physical play. Aside from humans, the animals that play the most are monkeys and apes, rodents, canids (dogs and wolves), felids (cats), elephants, and cetaceans (whales, dolphins, and porpoises). It seems that creatures need lots of playtime to develop "wild justice."

Self-handicapping is one of the most amazing illustrations of moral behavior in animal play. It occurs when a larger animal deliberately holds back while sparring with a smaller opponent. We call this a *moral* behavior because the larger animal cares more about both players having fun together than it does about winning.

Stuart Brown tells an amazing story in his book *Play*. He recounts how one time, in northern Canada, a hungry polar bear came upon a sled dog. The owner feared that his dog would become the bear's lunch, but, to his amazement, the dog settled into a "play bow" by extending its front paws and lifting its hind end. This posture is a common example of canine body language that signals, "I want to play with you." Incredibly, the polar bear accepted the invitation; it approached the dog in a zigzag line, signaling back that it was ready to play, rather than charging in a straight line to attack. Instead of killing the dog, the bear played with it for an hour, all while holding back its vastly superior strength. It even came back the next day to play with the dog again.

The sad ending to this story is that eventually the polar bear did revert to being a predator and killed the sled dog—surprising the humans who expected to see more interspecies wrestling. Perhaps their mistake was thinking that a few episodes of play would somehow transform prey and predator into friends rather than just unlikely temporary playmates. It was an understandable mistake, because in humans, of course, this is the very essence of how we become friends.

Brown makes a strong case that roughhousing prevents violent behavior rather than causes it. He writes, "rough-and-tumble play in animals and humans . . . is necessary for the development and maintenance of social awareness, cooperation, fairness, and altruism. Its nature and importance are generally unappreciated, particularly by anxious parents, who often see normal rough-and-tumble play behavior not as a state of play, but a state of anarchy that must be controlled." Brown goes a step further, linking rough-and-tumble play to the ability to control one's aggression: "Lack of experience with rough-and-tumble play hampers the normal give-and-take necessary for social mastery and has been linked to poor control of violent impulses later in life."

In other words, when we roughhouse with our kids, we model for them how someone bigger and stronger holds back. We teach them self-control, fairness, and empathy. We let them win, which gives them confidence and demonstrates that winning isn't everything. We show them how much can be accomplished by cooperation and how to constructively channel competitive energy so that it doesn't take over. We trust them, show them that we are trustworthy, and coach them on trusting themselves. These form the points of a healthy moral compass, which will serve as their guide when they leave home and enter the world.

Roughhousing Makes Kids Physically Fit

The physical-fitness benefits of roughhousing, for parent and child, don't require much explanation. To see for yourself how it beats a trip to the gym, just try SEAL (page 168) or Cat Leap (page 170), two of the more physically demanding and challenging activities in the book. Still, there are a few subtler points we'd like to make. Physical fitness isn't just about body strength; it requires complex motor learning, concentration, coordination, body control, cardiovascular fitness, and flexibility. Some of our moves require extreme concentration and strength, whereas others demand coordination and flexibility. Don't worry. Neither you nor your child has to be in perfect shape to get started. Find your limit and help your children find theirs, and then push that limit ever so slightly the next time you do the move together. You'll find that not only will the move take on new life, your bodies will, too.

Remember that not all physical activity is created equal. In *Recess*, Pellegrini explains why gym class and recess don't offer the same benefits. Both allow kids to run around and let off steam, but, because of the importance of free play, only recess leads to improved school performance and better social relationships. Remember that point as your roughhousing playtimes transition from set moves to improvisation—improv roughhousing is a close cousin to free play at recess (with the added benefit that no one is left out or picked on).

Roughhousing Brings Joy

By now, you can probably tell that we are total believers in play. If you're already a roughhouser, you don't need research to convince you that romping around is fun for both parent and child. Yet even we were surprised to learn that the fun and joy of roughhousing is hard-wired into our brains.

In *Affective Neuroscience*, Panksepp explains that the brain has circuits dedicated to various tasks: language, memory, attachment, assessing danger, and (of course) play. He found that when the play circuits of mammalian brains are activated, especially by roughhousing, the result is joy. Any activity that brings joy is considered to be hardwired into the brain. That's why rats will learn how to run a maze, even if there's no food at the end, as long as when they get there there's a chance to roughhouse with another rat. Bekoff and Pierce summarize the research well: "Play is not only serious business, but also fun. Animals get deep joy and pleasure from playing alone or with friends."

Brown notes similar behavior in otters, who are well known to play just for the fun of it:

> *One biologist who studied river otters decided to train some of them to swim through a hoop by offering a food reward for completing the task. Shortly after the otters learned to do this, the animals started introducing their own twists. . . . They swam through the hoop backward and waited to see if they got a reward. They swam through and then turned around and swam back the other way. They swam halfway through and stopped. After each variation, they waited expectantly to see if this version of the task would earn a reward or not.*

The otters were clearly eager to play for its own sake, not just to get food. And, in this playful way, they learned much more about how the world operates than if they had done the exact same trick for their food each time.

Roughhousing Has a Host of Benefits for Adults, Too!

Roughhousing develops young brains, but adult brains need workouts, too. Here's Stuart Brown again: "Our brains don't stop evolving after our twenties. Play very likely continues to catalyze neurogenesis [growth and connections of nerve cells] throughout our lives. . . . Dementia studies suggest that physical play forestalls mental decline. . . . Studies show a relationship between continued use of puzzles, playful exercise, games, and other forms of play and resistance to neurodegenerative disease." So there's yet another good reason to get off the couch and roughhouse—it might prevent Alzheimer's!

In fact, all the benefits of roughhousing apply to us as well as to our children, from boosting our emotional intelligence (as we tune in to our kids) to practicing empathy and moral judgment (as we hold back our strength and let our kids bowl us over). Active physical play is the best way for parents and children to build a strong, close, lasting bond. Obviously, this attachment is good news for kids, but it's even better news for grown-ups, especially dads, since many of us didn't get enough of that closeness when we were young. As dads, one thing we love about roughhousing is that it starts with physical activity but also stretches us in less familiar areas, like feelings, closeness, and intimacy.

One dad told us that he would often go with his son to "places [like woods and marshes] where we could be silly without being self-conscious." Getting filthy with sand and dirt was part of the fun, and he said that this kind of wild play was "a great cure for the grumpies." This dad recognized that play can be deeply meaningful, too. "When we would go puddle- or dust-jumping, or screaming, or singing, we sometimes talked or sometimes we didn't say a word. But there was never an empty silence between us—there were just times when we didn't need to fill the space with words."

CHAPTER 2

Get Started with Instant Roughhousing

"Do not be too timid and squeamish about your actions. All life is an experiment. The more experiments you make, the better. What if they are a little coarse, and you may get your coat soiled or torn? What if you do fail, and get fairly rolled in the dirt once or twice. Up again, you shall never be so afraid of a tumble."

—Ralph Waldo Emerson

W e know you probably don't read instruction manuals. But this chapter is different. You'll want to read it before getting started, because here we share some key roughhousing principles that will help you master the art. Then we'll present some simple instant roughhousing activities to get you playing.

Closeness and Confidence Take the Gold and Silver Medals

When you master the art of roughhousing, you send a strong message to your children: *Your power is welcome here, this is a place for you to be strong and confident, I will keep you safe, and we will be closer and more connected than ever.*

Closeness is the great payoff of spending active playtime with your children. Confidence is what they develop when they can count on you being by their side. Look for every opportunity to build your child's confidence by encouraging her to be strong and powerful. A great way to do so is to *reverse the roles* when you play. Let your child be the strong one—the monster, the scary dog, the doctor giving the shot, etc.—while you exaggerate being fearful or clumsy and incompetent. This switch gives kids a chance to feel powerful and release their tensions through waves of laughter. When in doubt, fall over. Falling over is always good for a laugh and helps your child feel more confident, because it means they are not always the one who is smaller, weaker, and more helpless.

Ramp Up the Enthusiasm

Rambunctious play might look like a simple physical activity, but as Yogi Berra said about baseball, "95% of this game is half mental." We can sum up the mental part very simply: *Extra enthusiasm, extra energy, and extra exuberance.* When you bring these qualities to your roughhousing, physical play will always seem more compelling and exciting than TV programs or video games.

Pay attention to your own feelings, too. Are you nervous about getting hurt? Are you re-creating scenarios from when your brother used to beat you up? Do you feel exhausted and just want to lie down on the couch with your eyes closed? These feelings might be signs to take a break or lighten up your roughhousing. And if you know you're a competitive person, you may want to dial back some of your natural instincts. Handicap yourself so that the child can experience power and confidence.

It's Not Just for Boys

Almost all children love and benefit from roughhousing, but boys engage in rough-and-tumble play much more frequently than girls. Of course, many girls roughhouse and many boys don't. But, as Pellegrini observes, the average gender difference is so consistent that it is probably a combination of both hormones and socialization—that is, of nature *and* nurture.

Boys as a group tend to tease, shove, and hit more than girls, even when they're having fun and being friendly. That's probably because more direct ways to show affection with other boys are forbidden after age three or four, when they risk being teased for being unmanly. That such emotional expression is taboo illustrates why boys need their parents, especially their dads, to show them how to have physical contact that isn't aggressive, to cuddle as well as to wrestle.

Girls, meanwhile, are famous for what is called *relational aggression*: cruelty through gossip, dirty looks, or a cold shoulder. Stuart Brown calls "a 'mean' girl who operates by psychological intimidation and exclusion . . . the equivalent of a boy bully, both of which interrupt the flow of play. As with physical aggression, kids are hurt. But in a healthy situation, girls learn what constitutes going too far and are closer as a result."

Roughhousing can in fact help break this mean-girl pattern— whether your daughter is the target or the Queen Bee. Through rough-housing, girls learn to be more direct about their feelings. We don't mean that they'll start punching their friends instead of gossiping about them. But after active physical play, your daughter will be more likely to speak up for herself and stand up for her friends.

We believe that all children, boys and girls, benefit from rough-housing at home. So make sure your son knows that he has a secure home base and that he can always climb into your arms for a cuddle or a good cry if his body or his feelings get hurt. And make sure your daughter has a chance to test out her strength and power, so that she can step out into the world with confidence.

Lots of men back off from physical contact as their daughters ap-proach or reach puberty. Don't give up roughhousing (or hugs), though, because girls need their dads to teach them that there is great value in non-sexual physical closeness.

Tune In, Don't Swoop In

Dads are famous for "swooping in" on their kids when *Dad* is ready to play. We will swoop up our child, throw him in the air, get loud and bois-terous, and flip him upside down. Some children will squeal with genuine delight. Others will protest loudly, which can make a dad feel rejected and give up on playing. A third group of children hate swooping but tolerate it because they are so eager for playful contact with Dad that they'll take it however it comes.

The alternative to swooping in is *tuning in.* Take a look at your child before grabbing her for a super-flip or a ride through the air. Is she calm and mellow? Maybe you can sit next to her and share that mellowness a moment. Then, *slowly,* you can introduce a more rambunctious and physically active style of play. Wildness and physicality are great—that's what this whole book is about—but it works best when it doesn't take kids by surprise. Of course, some older children love the excitement and suspense of a game where they know that at some unexpected moment you are going to sweep them up and launch them into the air. But you still need to really tune in and see if they like this game as much as you think they do—or as much as you do. On the other hand, when you tune in, you just might find that your child needs bigger challenges and more exciting surprises.

Another part of tuning in is managing the level of stimulation. It's the parent's job to understand how much stimulation a child wants and needs, and to help keep things in that range. You can lower the stimulation level by speaking softly, moving slowly, and taking breaks between moves. Of course, you may also want to rev up the stimulation level by being noisy, fast, and wild. Watch your child's emotions and facial expressions to see if you're in the right zone.

Rev It Up Earlier in the Day

Too many parents make the mistake of roughhousing right before their child's bedtime or bathtime. There is a natural arc of active physical play, which starts with calmness, rises into activation, reaches a peak of super-excitement, and then winds down. Attempts to interrupt the flow with pleas (or threats) for your child to settle down will backfire. She will only escalate more, refusing to calm down until there is a huge meltdown or showdown. But these big upsets are easy to avoid. Just figure out how long it typically takes for that arc to play out—it's probably somewhere between thirty and sixty minutes. Make sure to leave that much time, plus a little more for a cushion, between when you start roughhousing and when you expect to settle down for dinner, bath, or bedtime. This rule of roughhousing might mean that you have to change your schedule, but you'll see the payoff right away.

All Children Are Born to Roughhouse

Roughhousing is for *everyone*—including children with special physical or emotional needs. In fact, rough-and-tumble play often can be exactly what a special-needs child requires to build closeness and confidence. Child behaviorist Peter Smith writes, "Children with autism, or Asperger's syndrome, are generally not very interested in pretend play and avoid much social contact. However, one form of social contact they do often enjoy are gentler forms of rough-and-tumble play, perhaps initiated by an adult." Depending on the child, you may need to adjust your intensity, but a limitation in one area does not make your kid a fragile flower in every other area.

Roughhouse with Caution (But Not Too Much Caution!)

Safe roughhousing comes from knowledge and practice, but despite our best precautions, accidents will occasionally happen. Kids' joints—mainly elbows, wrists, knees, and ankles—are prone to injury during roughhousing playtimes. Pay particular attention to these areas and protect them as much as possible. Roughhousing can also injure heads and necks, so take great caution when performing any move that involves these areas, especially if your child is an infant. Practice first before going live!

If your child bumps her head against a hard surface, you should seek medical attention if she seems dazed or confused or if she vomits (you'll also want to check on her in the middle of the night). When in doubt, call your physician, call 911, or go immediately to an emergency room.

Finally, beware of what we call abdominal sneak attacks. This is when your kid decides that he is going to jump directly on your belly. The spleen and pancreas are surprisingly sensitive to this kind of impact and can be seriously injured. You might choose to give your children what we call the Harry Houdini Warning (the legendary illusionist died from complications of a ruptured appendix after receiving an unexpected blow to his abdomen).

No Obnoxious Tickling

Especially not the way your big brother used to tickle you. A quick little tickle or light jab is fine, provided you let your child catch his breath before doing it again. Laughter is an involuntary reaction and does not necessarily mean that the tickling is fun for your child. See how much laughter you can get with a fake tickle, where you *almost* touch your child in ticklish spots, but not quite.

In addition, make sure to stay "above the belt." No punching, kicking, biting, scratching, hair pulling, pinching, or headlocks allowed. Limit yourselves to pushing, holding, and grappling. If a violation occurs, don't abruptly end the roughhousing, but rather review the rules, listen to what your child has to say, and then reengage when everyone is ready.

Follow the Giggles

If you do something that makes your child laugh, do it again. And again. This advice might seem obvious, but as an adult it's easy to tire of a joke before kids do. To bring out the giggles, act silly, lose your dignity, and fall over a lot. Improvisation is another great source of laughter. Follow the flow; be loud, wild, outrageous, and exuberant.

On the other hand, roughhousing is sometimes accompanied by *no* giggles at all. If your child seems "dead serious," with an edge of real anger, then stop. But if there's a sparkle in your child's eye, focused concentration, and beads of sweat, that is a sign that you and she are working on *mastery*. This is a wonderful form of play that leads to deep learning and great satisfaction, like when kids get the hang of the monkey bars, or they finally build a tall block tower that doesn't fall over, or they shoot baskets over and over from the same spot until they get a rhythm going.

Freeze the Action Frequently to Keep Things Smooth

Make up a code word that means "stop," and use it frequently during roughhousing so that your kid can practice revving up and calming down (silly code words like "banana cream pie" often work best). Freeze like a statue as soon as you say the word, and encourage your child to freeze with you. In most cases you should keep the freezes short, just enough time to catch your breath. Injuries and taking time to review the guidelines call for a longer freeze. At first you might have to gently hold your child still after you call out the freeze word, but over time they'll get the idea. Use a different silly word to mean "go."

Emotional First Aid Goes a Long Way

Be sure to pause your roughhousing for major, minor, and even imaginary injuries. An imaginary injury is usually a sign that a child has deep feelings he or she wants to express, and is looking for a safe way to do so. In the case of such injuries, don't counter with, "You're not really hurt!" Instead, just listen. And use Band-Aids liberally!

Similarly, be prepared for great roughhousing to sometimes end in tears or a tantrum. This is normal: Emotional safety and closeness allow children to show their deeper feelings. Take a break from roughhousing to listen and provide comfort. Children's tears and other strong expressions of emotion are their best ways of showing us their feelings. Instead of pushing them to stop these feelings as soon as possible, allow a full release of them, which will let children regain their best thinking and their happiness and will get them back to roughhousing in no time.

Secure the Perimeter

OK, your attitude is set and you're ready to roughhouse. Now take a minute to check out the environment for your playtime. Notice any sharp corners, loose rugs, valuable glass vases, ceiling fans, and other potential hazards. Take off jewelry, watches, or anything that might break or injure someone.

Many of the moves and games in this book are best performed on a soft surface, like a mat, carpet, or grass. Avoid tile, hardwood floors, and cement. We recommend mentally visualizing all of the more complicated moves first and practicing with a big pillow prior to engaging with your child.

Warming Up

Before we get to this chapter's moves, here is a quick, practical, step-by-step warm-up program that will help get your energy flowing and your mind in gear. You can do this prior to any roughhousing playtime. Try each move for a couple minutes or until you get the hang of it. Your child might grow impatient and leap to the full-on wrestling at the end of the list. That's great; just go back up the ladder and practice the other steps when you get a chance.

1. Stand facing each other, a foot or two apart, and take turns shouting, "Ha!" This interaction always gets everyone giggling and loosened up. It isn't exactly roughhousing, but it is high-energy, face-to-face fun.

2. Hold your hands in front of you, with elbows bent, a few inches away from your child's hands. Start moving slowly, in a circle or back and forth in a line, trying to feel the "force field" between your hands so that it almost feels like you are pushing or being pushed, even though there's no contact. Flow between leading and following each other. This is a wonderful way to practice tuning in.

3. Start in the same position as in step 2, but this time touch your palms, keeping your elbows bent. Gradually push harder and harder, but match your strength exactly so that neither person's body moves too far.

4. In the same position as step 3, add an element of competition by trying to move the other person off the mat or out of a real or imaginary circle on the floor. Keep elbows bent and try to avoid sudden shoves. Make it as much a dance as a competition.

5. Now, place a mat or soft surface (a folded bedspread, for example) on the ground. Get down on hands and knees next to each other, facing the same direction, shoulder to shoulder. Start to interact in slow motion, bumping into each other and flowing above and below each other, like dolphins at play.

6. Build on the move in step 5 by again adding an element of competition. Try to maneuver the other person flat on the ground.

At each step, pay attention to what you're feeling: Are you impatient to get to "real" wrestling? Are you worried about hurting your child or getting hurt yourself? Do you feel silly? Afraid you're not doing it right? Wistful that you didn't get to roughhouse this way with your own parents, or nostalgic because you did? All these feelings are great to discover within yourself.

Airplane

This timeless move works great with infants, but older kids love it, too. Lie on your back with your legs bent at the hips and knees at 90-degree angles; place your kid, belly-down, across your shins. Now move your legs (and your child) forward and back and side to side so that she experiences just enough weightlessness and unpredictability for it to be thrilling without losing her lunch.

Alcatraz

Let your kids put you in a make-believe version of "The Rock"—a prison built of couch pillows or an area defined by the edges of the living-room rug—and then make a daring escape, allowing them to round you up again and put you back in the slammer. Start by giving in easily and then make it increasingly harder for them to catch and drag you back behind bars. Use your imagination to spice up the game (weren't there sharks in that water?). Variation: Some kids prefer to be the dastardly escapees. In that case, make it progressively harder for them to escape as the game repeats.

Almost Gotcha

All you have to do in this chase-and-miss game is run after your child, attempt to seize him, and then miss catching him at the last moment. You'll get more laughs if you fall over dramatically and reach pathetically for his legs. Then stand up and do it all over again. Children may signal loudly and clearly that they want the game to end with a successful catch and snuggle; otherwise, the game ends with you giving up in loud despair.

Bodylock

This game involves holding your child loosely but firmly on your lap or in front of you, and then defying her to slip or squirm free from your grip. You can clasp your own wrists or elbows for a tight but safe hold. Boast extravagantly of your escape-proof bodylock ("You'll never get away from me!"), and then act shocked each time she manages to escape. Increase the strength of your grip with each successive game. For a variation, try it with a group of children; you'll notice that some kids like to get help from their siblings or friends, whereas others prefer to escape all on their own.

Booby Trap

Pretend your hand gets stuck on everything it touches (i.e., the ground, the table, your kid's leg). It's the child's job to pry your fingers off the object. Let him do so, but make him work for it. Once your last finger is free, immediately stick your hand to another object. Variation: Pretend your two hands are magnets that clasp anything between them—like your child's body.

Boom!

Instruct your child to tap you on the chest with a single finger. When she does, fall with a dramatic crash to the ground, howling in mock agony. Really lose your dignity and get her laughing. Say, "You'll never be able to knock me over again!" Then repeat the fall-over-and-go-boom routine until she gains more confidence. In fact, whenever you're in doubt about what to do, just fall to the ground with a dramatic crash.

Bucking Bronco

Babies love being bounced gently on a knee, with occasional surprise drops of a few inches. You can play this game with older kids by mimicking a rodeo ride. Place your child facing outward on your knee, hold him under the armpits, and lift your knee up and down. Buck up and down as if you were a bronco that just downed several gallons of caffeine.

Clumsy Piranha

Kids love dangerous animals, especially when they're not *really* dangerous. Put a puppet or sock on your hand and chase after your child, pretending that the puppet is a piranha (or other deadly animal) that is ferocious but comically incompetent. Stumble about and miss biting your "prey" at the last moment. (Maybe bite the chair instead and spit splinters out of your animal's mouth in mock surprise.) This game is particularly great for children who are figuring out how to handle their aggressive impulses.

Knock Your Socks Off

This game is fun with two people, but even more so with a group. All players sit on the floor in their socks, with legs stretched toward the middle. On "Go," players try to yank other people's socks off while keeping their own socks on. You can tuck stolen socks into your pockets, but owners can snatch them back and put them on again. It's harder than you think to put a sock on one foot while preventing someone from stealing the other. The game ends when everyone but one person—the winner—is barefoot.

Leaning Tower of Babbo

The name of this move refers to Italy's famous leaning tower, but we've changed "Pisa" to "Babbo" (Italian for "Dad") because you're going to be the tower. Invite your child to climb up your body. When she is waist-high, hoist her up a little and then pretend you're a leaning tower: Tip back and forth, walk on your heels, spin around a little. Finally, fall down in a dramatic crash, making sure to land underneath, not on top of, your child. Naturally, this can also be a Leaning Tower of Mamma!

Lumpy Cushion

If your child is sitting on a couch, pretend not to notice and sit lightly on top of him. Say, "Boy, these cushions sure are lumpy! Wonder what I'm sitting on." Draw out the suspense as long as possible until finally realizing the lumps are your child. If you're pushed off the couch as you try to sit, act humorously horrified that the sofa doesn't seem to want you to sit on it, but announce that you're going to keep trying anyway.

Nudge

Physical contact with infants is all about stimulating their senses. Place your little one on his back on a carpeted floor. Then use your head and face to gently nudge him around—no hands! Your hair and face will provide a lot of beneficial sensory stimulation. When he pushes back, exaggerate your response, first flying backward and then coming back for more.

Olympus Mons

The largest known volcano in our solar system is Olympus Mons on Mars. Sit with your child on a bed or couch. Pretend you're both on top of Mons and that the floor below is lava. Alternate fluidly between trying to push each other into the lava and engaging in dramatic rescues.

Roly-Poly Derby

Curl into a ball on the ground, wrapping your arms around your legs. Tell your child to do the same. Now roll toward a predetermined finish line, "accidentally" smashing into each other along the way.

Sumo Dead Lift

We call this move Sumo (as opposed to Romanian) Dead Lift because Sumo technique will protect your back as you lift with your legs. First, invite your child to lie facedown on the floor. Then crouch, scoop under her torso and legs, and lift her up, Olympic-dead-lift-style. Once she's high above you, fly her around the room, making a soft bounce-landing on the couch or a gentle glide onto the floor. Throughout the lift, your points of contact should be her torso and legs. You can vary this move by acting like a forklift, with your child in front of you instead of over your head. Pretend she's a pallet of melons that mustn't get bruised ("Oops, crash, there they go!") or a sleeping python that suddenly wakes and starts slithering in your arms.

Wheelbarrow

This classic move needs little explaining. With your child in a push-up position (palms and stomach on the floor, legs extended behind), grab his ankles from behind, lift, and away you go! Set up cushions and towers of pillows around the house for crashing into. Scattering prizes for your child to grasp with one hand while on the move will build strength and coordination.

Zany Jazz Riff

This final instant roughhousing move was inspired by Sun Ra, one of the pioneers of free jazz. We love this guy because he claimed to be from Saturn, and his music made you believe it. In Zany Jazz Riff—which is basically free-form, improvisational roughhousing—the rules, tempo, energy level, and moves evolve as you and the children play together. It's never clear who's leading or who's following. You might start by getting down on all fours and daring your child to tackle you. Or dance through the house banging wooden spoons on pots. Or see if you can ascend a staircase without using any hands or feet—just like they do on Saturn. Go wild!

CHAPTER 3
Flight

"For once you have tasted flight, you will walk the earth with your eyes turned skywards, for there you have been and there you will long to return."

—Leonardo da Vinci

A   nthony's daughter Ava went through a Mommy-only stage at age three. Every night, around the end of dinner, she would announce that "only Mommy!" could put her to bed. If Anthony insisted on being involved, her demands intensified or escalated into a full-scale meltdown.

So one night, he tried a different approach. He invited Ava to journey with him through "The World of Flying Machines." Each night, Anthony would transform into a different flying machine (airplane, hot-air balloon, jet pack) and "fly" Ava up the stairs for bedtime. She loved the ritual, and after a few trips, Daddy's exile from bedtime vanished.

Banished parents can feel rejected and may want to give up on playing, but by sharing the excitement and closeness of their flying machines, Anthony and Ava were able to blast off in a new direction, one that built connection instead of disconnection. And once Anthony was welcomed back into the bedtime rituals, he realized that when Ava said, "Go away, Daddy," she was really saying, "I missed you, and I'm not quite ready to forgive you yet for being gone all day." So now, when Ava demands "Mommy only," Anthony answers, "I missed you, too. How shall we fly together tonight?"

All that flying up and down the stairs of the DeBenedet house built trust as well as closeness, and that's why we chose Flight to begin our in-depth exploration of roughhousing. Our flight moves are all about teaching trust: Trust yourself, trust others, and trust gravity!

Of course, for your child to learn trust, you must first *be trustworthy*. Whatever goes up must come down, so make sure you're standing by with arms outstretched. What's more, during flight moves, you must be emotionally attuned to your child so that you can distinguish the subtle differences between excitement and fear. Panic can sometimes resemble delight, so pay attention, check facial expressions, and learn exactly what your child likes best.

Flight moves also provide vestibular stimulation, a necessary component to healthy brain development that we often take for granted. The vestibular system—a labyrinth of spiral-shaped, nerve-filled caverns in our ears—is the epicenter of athletic prowess. It gives us the sense of where we are in space, how we got there, and where we're headed next. As fluid travels through these caverns during twirls or upside-down movements, we develop coordination, rotational and linear acceleration skills, and agility; it is by this process that your mind learns what it will feel like when your body twists or moves quickly during athletic activity. Physical and occupational therapists have long used gentle flight moves to help less-coordinated kids catch up with their peers; it's also helpful therapy for adults to address conditions such as dizziness and unsteady walking.

You already know hanging upside down and zooming through the air is a blast. Now you know it's good for the brain, good for attachment, and good for trust. So grab your cape. It's time for liftoff!

Essential Flight Skills

Lifting: The best way to lift kids is via their armpits. You can also lift children from their torsos—a hug-lift of sorts. Save upside-down ankle lifts for kids who weigh less than 50 pounds, because a greater weight can cause significant strain on their knee and/or ankle joints. In tray-lifts, the child's arms are bent and locked as if holding a tray, and you lift from underneath your child's locked elbows. Another safe option is the forklift, in which you use both arms to scoop-lift from underneath your child's back or belly. We advise against lifting children by their hands with their arms extended, because you risk dislocating their elbow joints. To protect your own back, always bend your knees before a big lift.

Twirling: The key to twirling is to establish a solid anchor. Anchors are the points of physical connection between you and your child. For twirls below the level of your head, armpits or hips/thighs work best. With an armpit anchor, your child's legs face away from you; with a hip anchor, your child's head faces away from you and her legs wrap around your waist. As the speed of your twirl increases, armpit anchors usually progress to arm/hand anchors and hip/thigh anchors progress to ankle/feet anchors (i.e., you'll naturally move your grip from your child's hips/pelvis to his thighs and, eventually, his ankles). If you're twirling your child horizontally above your head, make sure you have two secure anchor points—usually chest/armpit and inner thighs are best. Kids can be upside down or right side up for virtually all twirls.

Suspension: Suspension is a technique that emphasizes the few seconds of joy or suspense—before gravity takes over—that your child experiences when she is high above you or hanging upside down with only a minimal anchor, like an armpit or a leg. You can incorporate suspension into almost any flight move; just make sure it causes delight, not panic.

Release and Catch: When releasing your child from a flight move, he should be upright, unless you're releasing him horizontally from a forklift onto a bed or other soft surface. Advanced releases involve twisting or spinning your child in the air as part of the release. When you catch your child, concentrate on his armpits and torso. Never try to catch him via his extremities (hands, legs, or feet). Advanced catches involve *not* catching your child all the way, but rather aiding or slowing his downward descent using your arms/hands on each side of his torso.

Spotting: You don't have to be a gymnastics coach to understand the basics of spotting. To spot is to keep a person free from injury by gently helping her to a safe landing or guiding her through the completion of a move. The spotter does not catch the other's full weight but aims to keep the person upright, protect the head and neck, and absorb some of the shock of a fall. The key is to focus on the three Bs: your child's belly, back, and butt. To spot, place one hand softly on or just behind/below the most appropriate "B" spot. Your other hand should be upright in the air (as if you were taking an oath), ready to assist when needed. Most often, you'll only be providing an extra layer of confidence, but always keep your hands up and your knees bent in a springing position to help support any weight from a sudden slip or fall.

Balboa

Ages:	1 to 3
Difficulty:	Easy
Essential Skills:	Suspension, Release and Catch

Honoring Sly Stallone's famous fist pump in the Rocky movies, this move uses suspension to the max. Lift your child over your head via her armpits, then let go with your left hand and pump her up even higher by stretching the right—locked underneath her armpit—sky-high ("Yo, Adrian!"). When you're at the peak of your pump, make sure your child's center of gravity is nearly the same as yours; otherwise, you risk losing your anchor underneath her armpit. She will remain suspended until you slowly lower your arm. As she comes down, quickly place your left hand underneath her opposite armpit, release with your right, and pump back up again. If you've been training on the steps of the Philadelphia Museum of Art, you can run while your child is suspended or release her for a short free flight at the peak of your pump (almost like a shot put) before catching her with both hands on her return to earth.

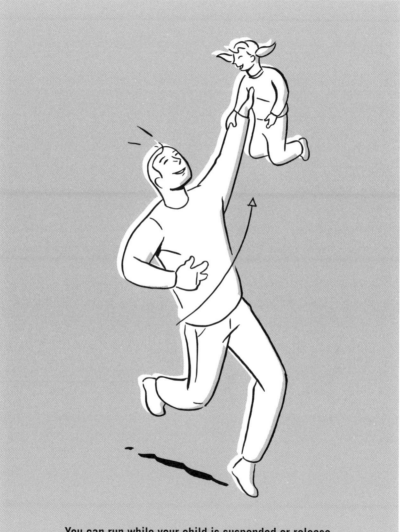

You can run while your child is suspended or release
her for a short free flight at the peak of your pump.

Rogue Dumbo

Ages:	2 to 5
Difficulty:	Easy
Essential Skill:	Twirling

In this move, the two of you will work together to mimic the actions of a wild, rampaging elephant. Lift your child, facing you, into your arms, with his legs around your waist, and then tilt his head and shoulders backward. When he's perpendicular to you, tuck his legs under your arms and allow your hands and arms to support his head and spine. He should now be hanging upside down, as if you are an elephant and he is your trunk. For the full effect, go rogue by twirling, swaying, snorting, trumpeting, and spinning around the house. With a little practice, your child can hang face-down, allowing Rogue Dumbo's trunk to be extended by the length of his outstretched hands.

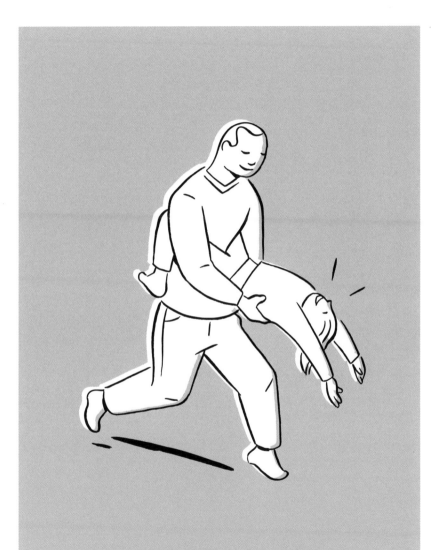

The child should hang upside down, as if you are an elephant and he is your trunk.

Sleeping Bat

Ages:	2 to 8
Difficulty:	Medium
Essential Skill:	Suspension

Stand face-to-face with your child. Hold his hands or forearms and direct him to walk up your legs and torso until he is horizontal. While you maintain your grip, have him arch downward and away from you until his head is at your ankles, facing away from you, and his legs are in front of your chest. (If he's older, he might be able to wrap his legs around your neck and shoulders.) You can swing your arms from side to side for added effect. Hold the position for a maximum of one minute. To end the move, have him flip his legs and feet away from your body while you maintain your hold on his hands or arms until he lands on the floor.

Although you may be able to suspend him longer than a minute, and some people (and bats) hang upside down for hours, doing so can cause unhealthy changes in your child's blood pressure. Not to mention that your arm muscles could quickly fail if you aren't used to isometric holds.

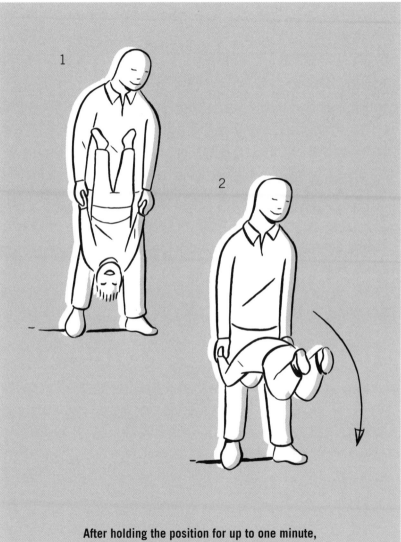

After holding the position for up to one minute,
have him flip his legs and feet away from your body.

Flying Fox

Ages:	2 to 7
Difficulty:	Medium
Essential Skill:	Lifting

This move simulates the experience of a zip-line, known in Australia and New Zealand as a "flying fox." For the uninitiated, it is a cable fixed at both ends, with one end much higher than the other, forming an incline. Attached to the cable is a pulley with a handlebar from which a passenger hangs to ride from one end to the other.

Begin by standing shoulder-to-shoulder, with your child on your dominant side. Hold your dominant arm, palm up, in front of her and a little above her head. Instruct her to grab your hand with both of hers, as if she were grasping the handlebar of a zip-line. She should bend slightly and then lock her elbows. Next, you both start running. Once you've picked up speed, use your nondominant arm underneath to lift the rest of her body higher into the air. She'll feel as though she's flying through the trees.

After about ten strides, lower her to the ground while continuing to run. Then hoist her up again and repeat. Flying Fox is useful for soaring over or onto objects such as rocks, couches, or puddles; higher objects require the child to perform exaggerated leg tucks.

Caution: To reduce the risk of injury to the child, your back, or both, do not raise her more than three or four feet off the ground.

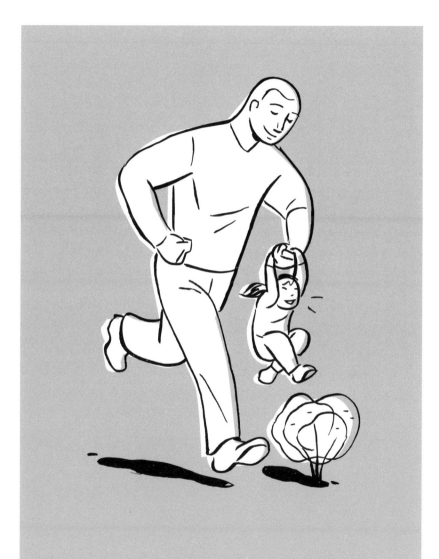

She'll feel as though she's flying through the trees.

Greek Catapult

Ages:	5 to 8
Difficulty:	Medium
Essential Skill:	Spotting

Since the Greeks invented the catapult, we named this move in their honor. Lie on your back and bring your knees to your chest, tilting your feet at a 45-degree angle. Have your kid crouch upright on your feet, facing away from your head and leaning forward, with his feet under his body. Now unbend and straighten your legs and, pushing your feet forward at roughly 30 to 45 degrees, catapult him forward into the air. Make sure you push your feet forward (rather than pushing them straight up) to prevent him from landing on you. He should land on his feet, a mattress, or a pile of soft pillows or couch cushions. A spotter is helpful for guiding the landing.

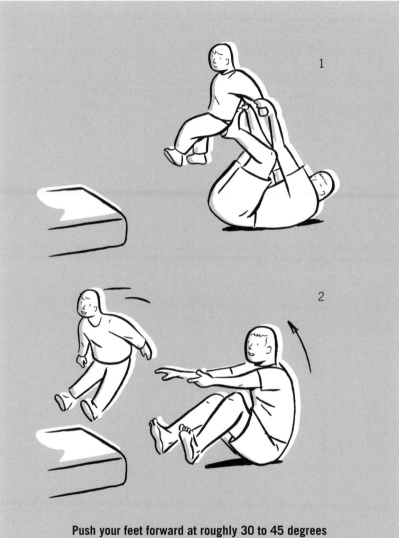

Push your feet forward at roughly 30 to 45 degrees
to prevent the child from landing on you.

The Balloonist

Ages:	3 to 6
Difficulty:	Medium
Essential Skill:	Spotting

Max Leroy Anderson, aka "Maxie," was born September 10, 1934, in Sayre, Oklahoma. He was an avid hot-air balloonist and in 1978 served as captain of the *Double Eagle II,* the first balloon to successfully cross the Atlantic Ocean. (In recognition of the feat, the crew was awarded the Congressional Gold Medal in 1979.) This move is our ode to Maxie, a celebration of this beloved ballooner's adventurous spirit as well as his contributions to the sport.

Begin on one or both knees. Invite your child to stand next to you on your nondominant side, slightly in front of you and facing across your body. Extend your nondominant arm in front of you, with palm up and elbow bent (as though holding a tray). Next, instruct your child to flip forward over your arm, using your dominant hand to spot her back. As she's flipping, guide her to land on your dominant shoulder (you'll need to dip it underneath her butt); she should be facing behind you. You'll be able to secure her well with just your dominant arm, but use your nondominant arm for extra support. This is the loading procedure to get your child into the "basket." Now stand up and begin jogging, occasionally crouching and then standing again, to simulate a hot-air balloon ride.

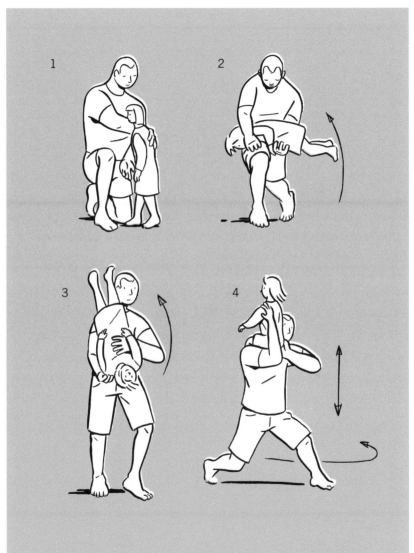

As she's flipping, guide her to land on your dominant shoulder.

X-15

Ages:	3 to 8
Difficulty:	Medium
Essential Skills:	Lifting, Spotting

Named after the fastest manned aircraft in history (it reached Mach 6.7), the X-15 combines a loading move, in which your child "boards the aircraft," with a "blastoff" that requires you to run as quickly as you can. To begin loading the aircraft, stand on your child's right side. Reach across her chest with your left arm while also reaching behind her legs with your right arm. Then lift and flip her, in one motion, onto your left shoulder so that she's lying horizontally, with her head pointed forward and arms outstretched (like wings). Place your hands under her armpits to secure her. Yell, "Blastoff!" and start running around, making crazy aircraft-engine noises and sonic booms. For a variation, hold your child with your left arm wrapped around her torso and your right hand under her chest. On a hot day, an epic battle can ensue as two or more X-15s run around outside, with each kid-pilot holding a water cannon in out-stretched arms.

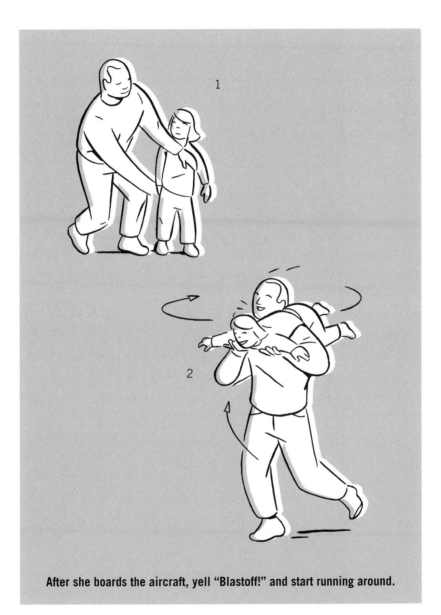

After she boards the aircraft, yell "Blastoff!" and start running around.

Acroyoga

Ages:	5 and up
Difficulty:	Hard
Essential Skill:	Spotting

Acroyoga is a form of partner yoga that incorporates acrobatics to facilitate trust and connection between two people, a base (you) and a flyer (your child). Even if you and your child are master yogis, we highly recommend using a third-party spotter. (It's a great opportunity for both parents to join the fun.)

Lie on your back and raise your legs together, bending at the hip to form as near a 90-degree angle as possible. Bend your knees slightly. With the spotter's help, your child should lie flat (belly-down) on the soles of your feet, with his head pointing in the same direction as yours. Separate your feet slightly to the outside of his waist/hips. Slowly straighten your legs and direct your child to extend his arms and legs, as though flying. The spotter should help with balance. You'll notice this move is similar to Airplane (page 35), except you're not holding onto your child and your legs are extended farther into the air. As a variation, the spotter can tilt your child downward so that you're almost face-to-face, forming approximately a 30-degree angle at your feet. Hold your child's forearms over your head so that his hands almost touch the ground. With the spotter's help, have him try a dismount by somersaulting over your head.

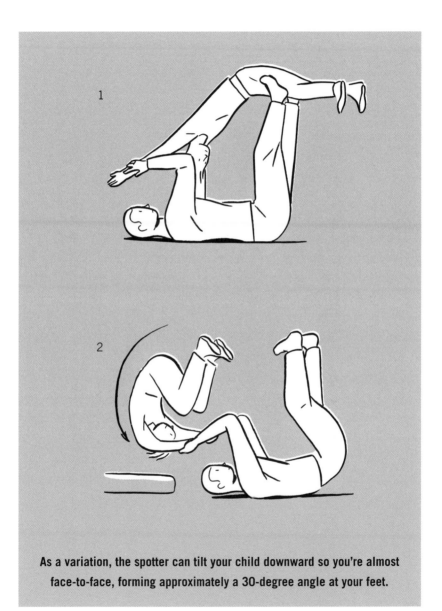

As a variation, the spotter can tilt your child downward so you're almost
face-to-face, forming approximately a 30-degree angle at your feet.

Human Cannonball

Ages:	5 and up
Difficulty:	Hard
Essential Skills:	Release and Catch, Spotting

When she was just fourteen years old, Rossa Matilda Richter, nicknamed "Zazel," achieved fame as the first person to perform the stunt of the Human Cannonball. The trick was developed in 1877 at the Royal Aquarium in London, and Zazel later toured with the P. T. Barnum Circus. This move allows your child to blast off like a human cannonball and then land safely on a soft mattress.

Begin by placing a mattress on the floor. Next, lie on your back, extend your arms in a T with palms facing up, and place your feet flat on the floor, bending your knees. Your toes should touch (or come close to) the edge of the mattress. Invite your child to stand barefoot on your hands and, leaning over your torso, place his hands on your knees. Next, he should bounce gently up and down in your hands. When you're both ready, count 3-2-1 and then launch him (at approximately a 45-degree angle) over your knees and into the air, adding a loud "Boom!" on blastoff. The child should do a side flop onto the mattress. Depending on his age and experience, you might want to practice his landing skills a few times before firing the cannon.

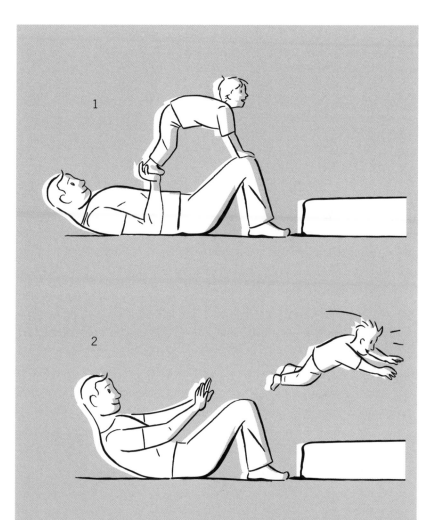

When you and your human cannonball are both
ready, launch him over your knees and into the air.

Wacky Whirling Dervish

Ages:	3 to 7
Difficulty:	Hard
Essential Skill:	Twirling

Sufi spinning is a form of meditation that consists of twirling one's body in circles for hours. But don't worry, this activity lasts only a minute or two. You'll need a smooth surface (such as a hardwood floor) and your child must be wearing socks for slipping; you should be either barefoot or wearing shoes for traction. Invite the child to lift his arms straight above his head. Stand in front of him, hold his hands, and step back a little, effectively tilting him forward at a 45-degree angle. Now begin twirling in a circle. At first, his feet will just slide around the floor, but as your speed increases, his feet will naturally lift into the air. For a fun variation, remove the child's socks and allow him to hang upside down from your body; he should wrap his feet around your neck while you support him from underneath with your hands while twirling. Stronger children will want only their feet to act as the anchor, but you should always provide back support.

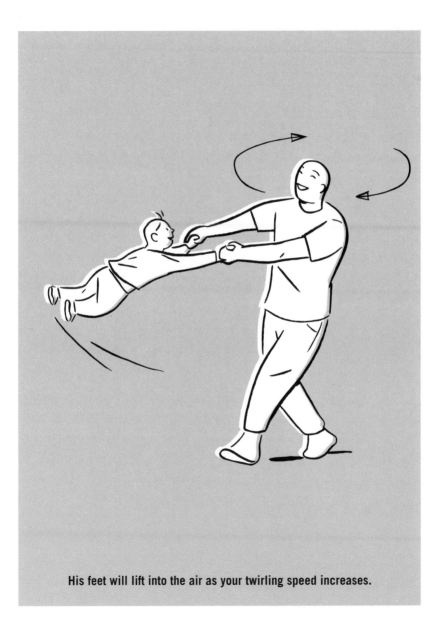

His feet will lift into the air as your twirling speed increases.

Real Stories from the Cockpit

We've heard many adults say, "I hated when my dad threw me up in the air, but I never told him, because it was so rare for him to play with me." Jerry was well on his way to being one of those dads. He was definitely a swooper. When he came home from work, he would run over to his daughter Kim and swoop her up, swing her in his arms, toss her in the air, and dance wildly with her around their apartment.

The only problem was, almost every time he did this, Kim screamed her head off. Jerry's wife, Pam, fussed at him, but he wasn't going to give up playtime with his daughter. When the conflicts between Pam and Jerry about these over-the-top antics got out of hand, the couple went to Larry for help. The solution was simple. First, Jerry changed his work schedule to be home sooner, to play *before* bedtime, and to finish his work after Kim went to sleep. That gave them a full hour or more for playing, which was (usually) enough time for Kim to get revved up and then wind down before bath and bed. As a bonus, Jerry and Kim got to enjoy some of that quieter time together, too.

More important, Jerry learned to tune in first, before introducing his flight plans. He sat down next to Kim when he got home, taking in whatever she was doing. After sitting with her a few minutes, building trust and closeness, he asked her if she wanted to fly. She couldn't yet talk well, but she almost always nodded eagerly and put out her arms, signaling for Jerry to pick her up. She loved a variation of Rogue Dumbo (page 48) that Jerry devised for her. He held her so that she lay on her back against his outstretched forearms, where she could look into his eyes. Then he cradled her head in his hands and swung her back and forth in front of him. As Kim got older, all that flying translated into a trusting relationship and a bold approach to life.

This story of Jerry, Kim, and Pam demonstrates that flight moves are wide open to variation. Don't hesitate to improvise. As Miles Davis, the great jazz trumpeter, said about improvisation: "Do not fear mistakes; there are none." You can improvise any flight move by adding the sound effects of jet fighters, hot-air balloons, birds, rockets, or screaming passengers. Suspension, one of the essential skills of flight moves, especially lends itself to improvisation. Every child is different when it comes to suspension, and a big part of successfully using this skill is knowing how to read your child. Does she like zero suspension (that is, being fully supported throughout a flight move), brief suspension (a millisecond), or long suspension (up to a couple of seconds of free fall or hanging upside down)? Remember that not every squeal is a sign of delight; the body reacts to a thrill even if the mind hates it, like laughing when you're tickled against your will. So start with no suspension, add a tiny bit at a time, and take in the feedback from your child.

When children are acting in an obnoxious or uncooperative way, one of the first things we need to do is attract their attention. That can be difficult, because the usual ways, such as screaming, can lead to new problems. Flight moves can be especially useful. A surprise launch into the air is an excellent way to get a child's attention without hits, screams, or threats. Playfully sweeping him into the air will "jiggle things up" and change the situation. (This technique is different from swooping in, which involves disturbing a completely calm child.) The goal is to capture his interest, not traumatize him.

Patty Wipfler, founder of Hand in Hand Parenting, calls this technique *the vigorous snuggle*, and she describes it as an extremely useful alternative to yelling, punishing, or ignoring misbehavior. Let's say a child refuses to clean up a mess. You can give her a couple chances, but if she digs in her heels and says, "No, I won't!" there's no need for threats or consequences. Just sweep her into your arms, snuggle her close, and with a big smile say, "Oh yes you will!" Fly her around the room, using her hand as a pretend magnet or vacuum cleaner that picks up toys and carries them back to the toy basket. The big smile and snuggly-fun aspect are key. These actions aren't designed to terrify children into submission but to snap them out of their "stuck" place. They reinforce the parent-child relationship, instead of knocking it down.

One day, during a rousing episode of Wacky Whirling Dervish (page 64), Tyler was twirling his son Davy through the air while they gripped each other's forearms. Davy bumped his foot lightly into a table leg, and although Tyler was pretty sure Davy wasn't hurt, the boy demanded a bandage. Tyler refused, insisting there was no cut or even a scrape. Davy grew upset, and at that point Tyler felt stuck because he didn't want to give in.

Tyler left his son crying on the floor for a minute to consult with his wife, who rolled her eyes a little and said, "Just give him a bandage, for heaven's sake. What's the big deal?!" Tyler was about to insist that bandages were only for blood, but he realized how absurd that sounded. He also realized he had narrowly escaped an I-told-you-not-to-play-so-wild-indoors lecture from his wife, so he hurried back to his son and said, "Let's pick out a bandage for you."

Between sniffles, Davy agreed, and together they headed to the medicine cabinet. Tyler decided to make it part of the fun, and they both came out of the bathroom covered in bandages. They rushed into the room where Mom was reading, shouted, "We're the Band-Aid Bandits," stole her book, and took off running. Tyler held his son around the middle while "Band-Aid Boy" held the stolen book in his outstretched arms. Mom chased them, and they all had a tremendous time. Since then, Tyler has dropped his rule that bandages are only for "real" injuries, because he discovered their symbolic healing powers, not to mention how useful they are as a superhero fashion accessory.

CHAPTER 4

Games

"Life is not a spectator sport. If you're going to spend your whole life in the grandstand just watching what goes on, in my opinion you're wasting your life."

—Jackie Robinson

One of the greatest roughhousing props is the mattress. On a bed, it's the quintessential trampoline; on the floor, the extreme mat. Bed jumping has the potential to go awry, but a little artful roughhousing can set things right again. A friend of Anthony's shared this story:

> *The other day I was jumping on the bed with my son Desmond. We were having a great time. Then we accidentally banged into each other; he fell off, cracked his head and leg, and started to scream. Desmond later calmed down and was OK, but at that point roughhousing was basically over in our house, especially anything that involved a bed and jumping. It was like that children's counting song, "No more monkeys jumping on the bed!"*

Anthony thought about his friend's experience. He understood the impulse to cut out the rowdiness but knew that bed jumping can be safe and fun. *Multiple people* jumping on a bed at once can be dangerous, however, and five little monkeys jumping on a bed is just asking for trouble. The *Art of Roughhousing* philosophy is that safety comes from knowledge, not from prohibition, so Anthony devised Ejection Seat, a one-person-at-a-time bed-jumping game, which you'll read about on page 84. After learning this move, Dad and Desmond rediscovered roughhousing, and there were no more incidents involving blood.

Games are the type of childhood play that most commonly continues into adulthood. The benefits of game-play also continue into adulthood and in fact are crucial for adult success. Games provide a playful introduction to competition. With roughhousing games, the primary task is to help children learn to welcome competition, instead of running from it or obsessing over it. Focus on fun, confidence, and skills, rather than on winning and losing.

Skills are built through repetition, so these roughhousing games are designed to be played over and over, for as long as the giggles or "serious fun" endures. Games also provide children with a balance between teamwork and individual accomplishment. The result is the ability not only to tolerate losing but also to be a gracious winner.

When Larry's daughter Emma was in fourth grade, they both dreaded violin practice. She was definitely not headed for the philharmonic, but Larry felt she needed to stick with it and put in the required practice time. After weeks of tears and arguments, they stumbled upon a solution. Whenever Emma got frustrated during violin practice (which was every single time), she and Larry played a game they called Smashup. Emma took a squishy ball and hurled it at the wall. Larry screamed in fake pain, as if it were his head that was crunching against the wall, rather than the ball. Emma laughed and threw the ball again.

Once Emma's frustration level lowered from the giggles and physical exertion of Smashup, they would thumb wrestle. The winner's prize was to choose five fewer or five extra minutes of practice. Either way, they made it through violin practice without any actual heads (or instruments) smashed, and Larry and Emma grew closer as well (instead of building up resentment and frustration).

More than any other type of roughhousing, games require coordination of three aspects of human intelligence: physical, social, and cognitive.

Physical intelligence refers to excellent motor skills. It might seem odd to consider physical skills as a form of intelligence, but think about how great athletes have such a keen knowledge of where their bodies are in space and how well they coordinate different parts of the body to do different things simultaneously. The fast and physical roughhousing games described in this chapter build all the elements of physical intelligence, including hand-eye coordination, quick reflexes, and good balance.

Social competence is a fancy name for street smarts or common sense, and games are a great way to develop it. Through games, we learn how to read other people, so we know whom to trust and whom to call on a bluff. We learn how to communicate and when it's best to hold our cards close to the chest. We learn how to anticipate and think a few moves ahead and how to make the most of a bad situation.

The most important social benefit of game playing is the way it helps children let go of the need to win every time or always be the best. To make friends and keep them—or just to keep a good game going—you have to be willing to follow the rules even if they don't go your way. You sometimes have to let other people decide which game to play. You can't be a sore loser or you'll quickly run out of people willing to play with you.

Which brings us to the single most frequently asked question parents ask about kids and games: Should I let my child win? We think the answer is yes—usually—because winning at home builds the confidence children need to play against their peers, who are certainly *not* going to let them win.

Ned's son Mark had to win every game at home—*or else*. Ned worried whether Mark would ever be able to play without being given an unfair advantage. One day, though, Ned took his son to the gym. Mark, then about nine years old, wanted to watch some teenage boys play basketball, so Ned left him there while he worked out. When Ned came back, Mark was in the game, and the boys weren't cutting the little kid any slack. They blocked Mark's shots, stole the ball from him, body-checked him on their way toward the goal. He was sweating, breathing hard, and had a serious expression on his face. Ned sat on the bleachers and watched. Mark gave his dad a quick smile and refocused on the game. His team lost. Ned waited for an explosion of tears and angry accusations, but that didn't happen. Mark went straight over to his dad (after high fives to the big kids on both teams) and said, "That was *really* fun." All that confidence-building at home had paid off.

We said that we *usually* let kids win—there are exceptions. When your child asks if you let her win or if you're playing your hardest, you can answer, "Would you like me to?" After they've won a million games against you, they may want to gain confidence by really testing themselves, even if that means losing. You can help move things in this direction by slowly increasing how hard you push them before they win or by winning occasionally when you play brief games (like Appel, page 76) again and again.

Anthony's daughter Ava used to make up her own rules to the game Memory, which resulted in everything going ridiculously her way. After a few games like this, Anthony started to ask her, "Would you like to play by the official rules, or would you like to play by Ava Rules?" Sometimes she chose real rules, because she wanted to see what a fair game was like, and sometimes she chose Ava Rules, because she wanted to fill herself with confidence and the certainty that life with Dad isn't a competition.

When children cheat at games, don't punish them; they're just trying to even out the playing field because they know they're smaller and less experienced than you. Let them know with a smile that you see what they're doing, but let them get away with it until they don't need to anymore.

Some parents, especially fathers, insist on pushing their children hard at home to prepare them for the harsh world outside. We disagree. Let the focus be on joy and closeness, even in competitive games. After all, lots of men complain that their fathers were too hard on them, but we've yet to hear a man complain of having too much joy and closeness from playing super-fun games with his dad.

In addition to physical and social development, roughhousing games contain a strong *cognitive*, or thinking, aspect. This benefit comes from the way children use simple games as stepping-stones to mastering increasingly complex games. The skills get tougher, the rules get more complicated, and the games take on layers of sophistication. That all takes a lot of brainpower. No wonder that, as Anthony Pellegrini discovered, children who are good at games are usually good at friendships, and well-liked children tend to be good at games.

Essential Game-Playing Skills

Physicality: Physicality is the main difference between roughhousing games and board games. All the games here have an element of physical contact. You can add physicality to virtually any game. Take the classic rock-paper-scissors: When rock beats scissors, you could swat the other person's scissors with your rock. Or if paper beats rock, you can give the rock a tight squeeze with your paper. Just make sure to match the intensity of the whacks and squeezes to what your child will enjoy.

Adventure: Create just the right sensation of adventure or danger to keep the excitement level elevated throughout the game. Adventure in a game can be imaginary or real (both will boost adrenaline). Some imaginary examples include lava, sharks, and quicksand; real examples include hills, woods, and balance beams.

Losing and Winning: Kids need a chance, with you, to build up confidence and mastery so they can confidently face the competitive outside world. Watch that your own competitiveness doesn't get out of hand, and let them win until they signal to you that they want you to step up your game.

Rules: Games have rules, and it's important to teach them to kids, but it's also OK to keep rules loose. You can adapt existing rules or even make up new ones as you play. Children love to argue about rules, so remember that's part of the fun. Just as you don't need to win every game just because you're bigger and stronger, you also don't need to win every argument about the rules, either.

Know-How: All games require practice of particular skills. Some children adapt easily to the idea that they need to work at perfecting their technique; other kids feel like giving up if they don't do it perfectly the first time. Let them see that you have to practice, just as they do. When games are fun and full of laughter, children are more motivated to keep practicing and develop their know-how.

Appel

Ages:	5 and up
Difficulty:	Easy
Essential Skills:	Physicality, Losing and Winning

Appel (pronounced *ah-PEL*) is a fencing term used to describe the stomping of one's foot to produce a sound that distracts one's opponent. Start your roughhousing-style duel by facing your child, with each of you stepping the left foot a few feet back. Stomp your right feet alongside each other, toes next to heels. Feel free to let out a "kee-ya!" Hold left hands or grasp each other's left forearms. You each can now move any part of your bodies except your planted right feet, and you must keep your left hands clasped. The first person to dislodge the other's planted foot wins. If one player is left-handed and the other is right-handed, alternate front feet for each bout. This game is fun to combine with a staring contest: Maintain eye contact throughout the duel, earning extra points if you're the last to smile or laugh, in addition to being the one to keep your foot immobile.

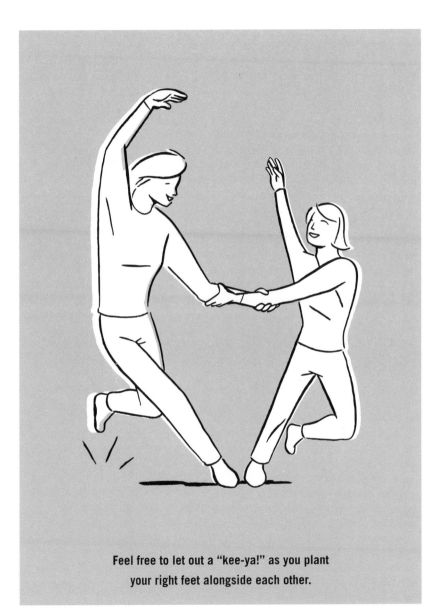

Feel free to let out a "kee-ya!" as you plant
your right feet alongside each other.

Raucous Pillow Fight

Ages:	4 and up
Difficulty:	Easy
Essential Skill:	Losing and Winning

The best pillows for whacking are the big, fluffy sleeping kind, rather than the small, hard sofa kind. When battling your opponent, always hold the zippered part of the pillow and whack with the other end to prevent injuries like eyeball lacerations. The best pillows for hurling are zipperless couch pillows. (Why do you think they call them *throw* pillows?) Older kids might like to have objectives, as in ten head whacks and five leg whacks result in a win. Younger children love when you fall over dramatically after being hit. Always match your strength to that of the child.

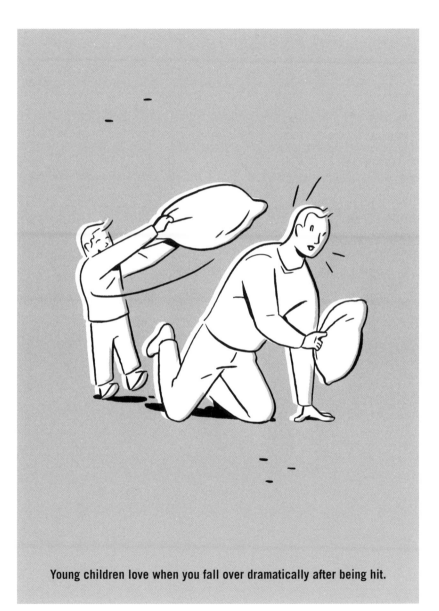

Young children love when you fall over dramatically after being hit.

Chariot Race

Ages:	4 and up
Difficulty:	Medium
Essential Skills:	Physicality, Losing and Winning

This game, named in honor of the most popular nonlethal spectator sport in ancient Rome, is best played outdoors on a large grassy area; it can be played indoors, as long as there's enough room for a course without the risk of crashing into walls. The course should be short to allow for multiple laps. It should also be narrow to maximize body contact, which is the source of most of the fun. In ancient times, riders gained the advantage by purposefully knocking opponents off their chariots, especially when making a turn. Here, players also try to knock one another down.

There are two main racing positions: One is bear-crawling on your hands and knees; the other is crab-walking on your hands and feet. Players can alternate positions with each lap. For the bear-crawling position, players can use only their shoulders to knock opponents down. For the crab-walking position, only hips can be used. If multiple adults and kids are playing, adults adopt the bear-crawling position and kids ride on the adults' backs. (Make sure to go outdoors for this one.) Remember that *you* should be the one getting knocked over most of the time! If this game becomes a favorite, consider wearing knee pads to avoid soreness and injury.

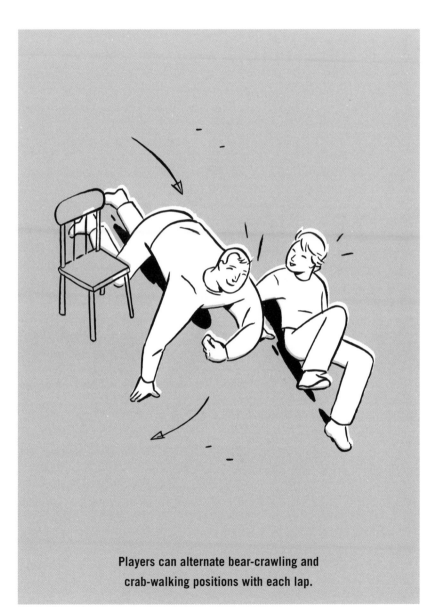

Players can alternate bear-crawling and crab-walking positions with each lap.

Cliffhanger

Ages:	3 and up
Difficulty:	Medium
Essential Skill:	Know-How

This game focuses on cooperation more than competition. First, assume the basic position: Bend at the hips and knees and squat as if sitting on a chair. Next, invite your child to stand on your thighs, holding your hands. Then incorporate the hanging aspect by letting go of one hand. Now she can lean back as though hanging from a cliff. When you're both ready, signal that it's time to switch hands in midair. A spotter is useful when first attempting this activity.

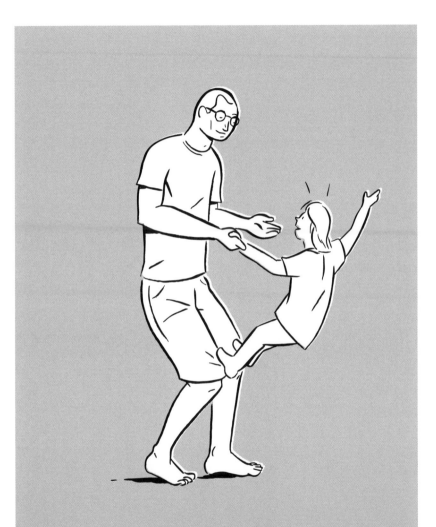

Incorporate the hanging aspect by letting go of one hand.

Ejection Seat

Ages:	5 and up
Difficulty:	Medium
Essential Skills:	Adventure, Know-How

In 1916, inventor Edward Calthrop patented the first aircraft ejection seat. His contraption used compressed air, whereas today's seats harness the power of explosives.

In this activity, you and your child will eject, one at a time, from doomed fighter jets. You'll need a bed that's in a room with wide, unobstructed floor space and a high (8-foot to 10-foot) ceiling. To play, one person bounces on the bed, building up height and momentum, while the nonbouncer makes fighter-plane sounds and then shoots the other person down, triggering the need to deploy the ejection seat. To do so, bounce as high as you can, bouncing your way toward the edge of the bed; drop to your butt, bounce once, and propel yourself forward off the bed. The person who goes the farthest wins. A tip for achieving greater distance: Plant your hands on the bed when you drop to your butt, then push off as you land. Curse you, Red Baron!

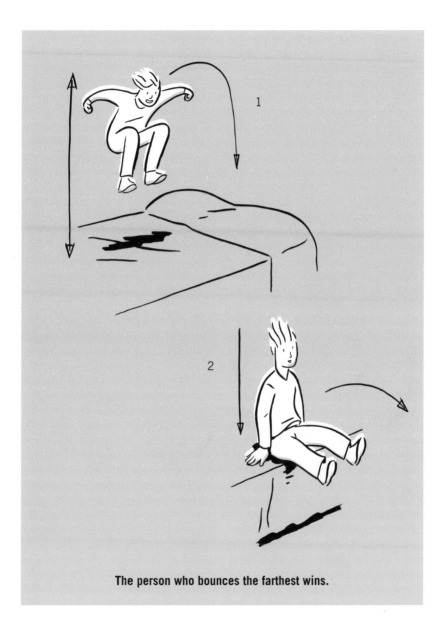

The person who bounces the farthest wins.

Full Squadron Water-Balloon Fight

Ages:	5 and up
Difficulty:	Medium
Essential Skill:	Losing and Winning

A couple things will take your water-balloon fight from run-of-the-mill to wicked fun. First, you need lots of kids, say, ten to fifteen. If the children are younger, plan the game with all their parents; if they're older, let your kids round up friends themselves. Second, prepare a lot of water balloons. That's where most water-balloon fights go awry—participants run out of ammo before energy levels wind down. We recommend 300 ready-to-launch balloons, which usually last about one hour for a squadron of fifteen. For added fun, construct a homemade launcher using a plastic funnel and bungee cords (or any available elastic materials). Each team should also have a "home base" containing a bucket (or comparable object) that opposing teams try to knock down with the balloons. Discourage head-hunting. (Winter variation: snowballs.)

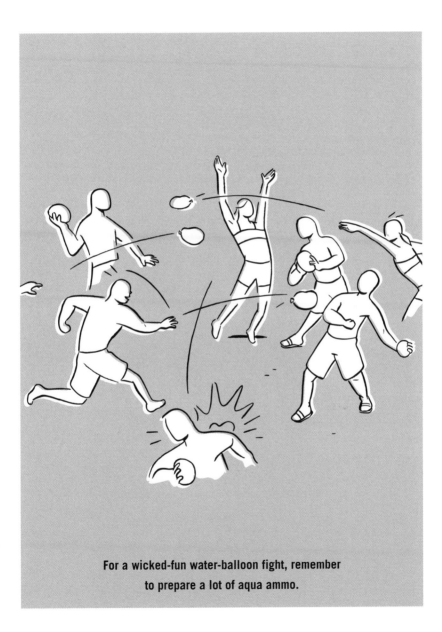

For a wicked-fun water-balloon fight, remember
to prepare a lot of aqua ammo.

Jousting

Ages:	4 and up
Difficulty:	Medium
Essential Skill:	Rules

The first-ever jousting tournament is reported to have occurred in 1066. The primary objective for jousting knights was to unhorse their opponents. The same is true for this game (minus the horses). You'll need a seven-foot two-by-four board and a couple pool noodles, which will serve as your lances. Start by elaborately challenging each other to a duel. You and your squire may don "armor," like gloves, hats, or coats. Lay the board flat on the ground and stand on it at opposite ends. Start poking at each other with the noodles until one person falls off. Try to avoid head swipes.

A cool variation (which we call Friar Tuck) involves only one noodle, which you both hold at opposite ends. Each person also has an object on the ground on opposite sides of the board. The goal is to keep one hand on the noodle and use the other to try to grab your object without falling off. Any clever child will discover that if she suddenly releases the noodle you will crash to the ground. Let her figure out this trick once and then issue a royal decree outlawing it.

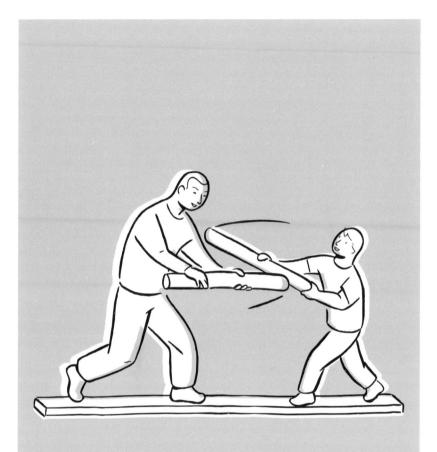

Joust at each other until one person falls off the board.

Vaquero

Ages:	7 to 12
Difficulty:	Hard
Essential Skill:	Know-How

The word *cowboy* first appeared in the English language in the 1700s; it was derived from the Spanish word *vaquero*, a person who manages cattle on horseback. In this game, you and your child will each get to play the steer and vaquero.

You'll need a rope that's at least 1/2 inch thick and 7 to 10 feet long; an athletic or "tube" sock; and a soft ball (e.g., a Nerf softball). Make your lasso by inserting the ball in the sock and tying the sock to the rope. The object of the game is for the vaquero to wrap the lasso around the steer's lower legs. When that occurs, the lassoed steer should cooperate and let herself be roped in. We recommend avoiding neck wraps, sticking to leg lassos only.

A fun variation for playing with multiple children: Direct the steers to form a circle around the adult vaquero. The vaquero swings the lasso in a wide circle just above the ground, and the steers jump over it. When a steer misses a jump and gets lassoed, the vaquero can reel 'em in!

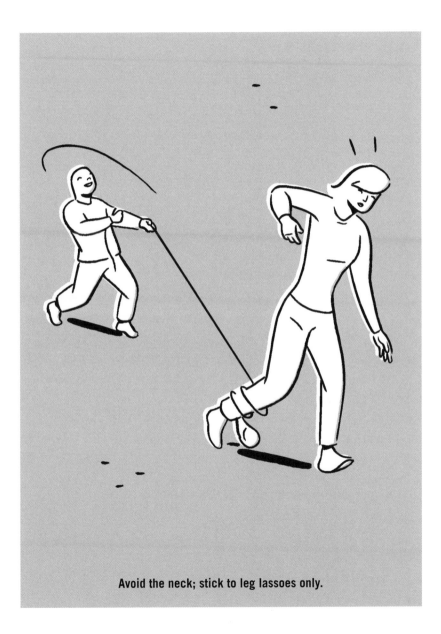

Avoid the neck; stick to leg lassoes only.

Real Stories from the Playing Field

More than a hundred years ago, the great Swiss psychologist Jean Piaget studied children at play; he was probably the first scientist to view games as a serious topic for study. He discovered that games teach children fairness, morality, and how to stick up for themselves and their friends. Believe it or not, he thought one of the most valuable aspects of childhood gameplay was the way kids argue about rules. He would surely hate the way most children's games nowadays are organized and refereed by adults.

Piaget may have valued children arguing endlessly about rules, but most parents dread it. If you're anything like us, you've shouted, "If you keep arguing about who's in and who's out, you won't have any time to play!" One day, Larry's daughter Emma and her friend Gabe were playing tag. Except they weren't actually playing. They had decided to play tag but were instead arguing endlessly about which type of tag to play. After Larry begged them for the tenth time to stop arguing and start playing, Gabe's father stepped in. He said mildly, "Hey, Larry, I think that arguing is the game they want to play." Leave it to the child psychologist to miss the obvious.

More than any other area of roughhousing, children experience tension about games. Some kids develop tension about the game's rules and the way those rules are enforced (probably because of adults who interfere too much). The best way to relieve this tension is to invent silly rules that the kids are allowed to break. Don't worry; this won't lead them to break important rules. In fact, it will help them cooperate with reasonable rules because, through roughhousing, they can release their rule-related tension.

We like to use Raucous Pillow Fight (page 78) for this purpose. You can get a great game started by saying, "OK, buddy, there's only one rule.

No bopping me on the head with this pillow, and I mean it!" Of course, your voice and facial expression convey that you don't really mean it, that you're just playing (just like the "play face" of rhesus monkeys and "play bow" of dogs and wolves, discussed in Chapter 1). The point is for the child to playfully defy the rule, bopping you good on the head. Then you take off after her in mock anger, remembering to keep it lighthearted and playful. You might add to the comic effect by tripping and falling just before reaching her, at which point you announce, "New rule! No hitting me with pillows when I'm down." As she clobbers you with pillows, you're building her confidence as well as your relationship. This game and the laughter it provokes provide release of tension about rules, which results in a child imbued with good ethics and morals, a child who follows rules because everything runs more smoothly when people act decently toward one another.

Chariot Race (page 80) is another activity that relieves tension about rules. As you and your child crawl around your homemade colosseum course, knocking each other over as you go, you can both make up new rules. Some will be imposed by your child, who is eager to win every time. He might declare that your shoes must be tied together or that you have to stay down for ten seconds after being knocked over. Your job is to go along with his rules while loudly (but humorously) voicing your objections. You can shout, "That's not fair!" as much as you want, but since it's roughhousing and you're self-handicapping (page 20), let the rule stand.

Some children develop so much angst about winning and losing that, as adults, they never grow out of it. Bo was a huge sports nut, but he was barely able to play because he couldn't bear to lose. For him, we made up the Winning and Losing Game, which we have since played with many other children. The idea is simple. You say, "Let's play the winning and losing game," to which your child asks what the heck you're talking about.

Explain that you've noticed he has trouble with winning and losing, and you want to play some games together to help him out. We call this process "bringing the problem onto the playing field." You can pause there to see if he has any good ideas for what a winning and losing game could be. If he doesn't, then it's up to you. When we play, we just toss a coin in the air, and one person calls "heads" or "tails." Whoever wins puts on a wild victory dance; whoever loses has a big fat temper tantrum ("You cheated! That's not fair!"). That's the whole game. Everyone giggles, and then you play again and again, for as long as it's funny for your child. This game does not promote bad sportsmanship. On the contrary, after the child releases tension about winning and losing through waves of laughter, he's able not only to better handle real defeats, but also to be more gracious about his victories.

Another tip for supercompetitive kids is to let them retain their competitive edge but build teamwork. You might ask them to pair up with a friend or sibling to take you down to the mat, so they can see how much stronger they are with a friend than on their own. You can also downplay the thrill of victory and the agony of defeat by giving out awards for style, gracefulness, effort, and sportsmanship.

Some children, meanwhile, develop lots of tension about the basic skills that games require. One boy started every playtime for a year with the words, "Go easy on me, I'm just a kindergartner!" He did fine as long as he was given the chance to gradually build up confidence. Other kids don't even get this far, because they give up after their first frustration or humiliation. The result is that they never develop the skills every child (and adult) needs, like throwing, catching, kicking, balancing, and running.

Parents can do a lot to help in this situation. The first step is to empathize with your child's feelings, saying, "It's really frustrating not to be able to do what the big kids can do. And it must have felt awful to be teased about it." Empathy is much more effective than telling your child to "get over it" or calling her names for falling short of your expectations. The next step is for you to miss the ball, fall, trip over your own feet, and get your child giggling any way you can so that she doesn't always feel like the bumbling incompetent one. If she teases you mercilessly about it, don't yell at her. She's merely passing on the humiliation she felt when she was (or feared she would be) teased. Your job is to take it in stride, maybe giving a fake "Waaah! You're teasing me just because I fell over. Oops, I fell over again!" If you turn it into a game, these feelings can dissipate without anyone getting hurt. Finally, you can help reluctant kids develop game skills by incorporating lots of high-energy fun whenever you play. Don't just run drills, unless your child happens to love drills. Instead, include lots of physical contact (like a big hug or high five) after every try. Incorporate basic skill building into roughhousing games, like using pillow fights to practice throwing and catching, or playing Cliffhanger (page 82) to improve balance.

When children play in groups, they often feel tension about being included or excluded. Adults can play an important role here, helping every child to feel part of the group. Let kids set and argue about the rules, for the most part, but insist that no one be left out, especially those who are prone to exclusion because they're smaller, less coordinated, disabled, or new to the neighborhood. You don't have to take over; just smile broadly and announce, "Everyone gets a turn" or "I'm going to help Joe because he hasn't had as much practice with this game" or "Latasha gets as many tries as she needs until she hits the ball."

A final source of tension surrounding games comes from children's fears about getting hurt and showing weakness. For a boy named Nils, Larry invented a game called the Designated Screamer, designed to help children handle their emotions when they get hurt rather than stoically toughing it out. When he was about seven years old, Nils was playing basketball and banged his knee pretty badly. He instantly got up and started playing again. Nils was clearly in pain, but he denied it and insisted on continuing. Having failed to convince him to take a break, Larry started jumping up and down, howling, "Ow! My leg is in extreme agony!" Nils asked him what was wrong. Between humorous howls of pain, Larry explained that, just as in baseball, which has a designated hitter, he was the "designated screamer" who would do Nils's screaming for him so he could keep playing. Nils, a big Red Sox fan, immediately got the joke and laughed even more at Larry hopping on one foot and making a fool of himself. Then Nils said he'd like to rest his leg a little before rejoining the game. That was a major accomplishment. Seeing Larry exaggerate his pain, without making fun of him, allowed Nils to overcome his fear of looking foolish (or "girlish," which some boys think is the worst thing in the world). Playing injured, which is a common trend in professional, college, and even high school sports, isn't manly; it's just dumb. Paying attention to an injury isn't a weakness; it's smart.

Like every form of roughhousing, games are wide open to improvisation. You can add the essential skill of *physicality* to any backyard sport by incorporating hugs and playful wrestles every time you tag your kid out in baseball or she scores in basketball. You can even turn a quiet indoor board game like Chutes and Ladders into a rambunctious roughhousing activity: Prop a big sofa cushion against the sofa; every time a player lands on a chute, he jumps to the top of the cushion and slides down. You can also improvise with the element of *adventure*. In Jousting (page 88), for example, you can add excitement by elevating the board with a few bricks.

We'll close this chapter with the story of Brandon, who month after month spent a fortune on tickets to take his three sons to professional sporting events. Every outing ended in disaster. The boys were bored, fought obnoxiously, and demanded endless souvenirs and concessions. Brandon yelled and threatened to stop taking them. The boys just shrugged their shoulders, which made him even angrier. One day Brandon's wife calmly suggested that, before buying the next batch of tickets, maybe Brandon should ask his sons if they would rather do something else during their special Daddy time. He was skeptical, but he tried it.

Turns out, when offered the choice, each child wanted to do something different with Dad. The oldest wanted to play sports at the park, not watch them from the bleachers. The youngest wasn't interested in sports at all, but he did want to roughhouse; father and son discovered they both especially liked wild pillow fights and anything that involved jumping on the bed. To Brandon's great surprise, his middle son wanted to go to games with him—he just didn't want his annoying brothers along. Once in a while, they would all go to a game, or pile on top of Dad in a free-for-all, or play a pickup game with other kids in the park. Brandon loved his one-on-one time with each son. Looking back, he had to laugh at all the times he dragged them along for "quality time" at the game.

CHAPTER 5

Contact

"Once you've wrestled, everything else in life is easy."

—Dan Gable, Olympic gold-medal wrestler

From rambunctious wrestling to wild flips and rolls, physical contact is the heart of roughhousing—and, really, at the root of our experience as humans. We are all social beings; we require connection with other people. If we're lucky, we exist in close, warm, loving connection, not isolated and alone. In every culture, healthy touch is the most basic way to communicate that connection. Once we reach the age of two or three, we also have words to express love. Yet nothing ever replaces the power of physical contact, because nothing else shows other people so clearly and so well that we are *really there* with them.

It turns out there are two types of physical contact that greatly impact people's lives. One is tender, such as rocking a baby to sleep. The other is playful, like rolling down a hill with your child tucked in your arms (see Steamroller, page 108). Both types activate our tactile sensory neurons. They also trigger brain circuits for pleasure, contentment, and joy, creating a lifelong link between healthy touch and positive feelings. Good physical contact instantly signals safety and connection by releasing the hormone oxytocin, sometimes called "the cuddle chemical." That's why we advocate beginning and ending all roughhousing sessions with hugs and high fives.

The chemicals that are released in our brains when we give or receive genuine touch don't just promote exuberance, delight, and happiness; they can be healing as well. The right kinds of touch can be soothing, calming, energizing, and therapeutic. Researchers have begun to explore the effect of affectionate touch between spouses on cardiovascular health, with the hypothesis that more touch leads to cleaner arteries. Like compound interest, good hugs build on one another, leading to overall greater happiness. When we're happier, we feel less stress—which is good for blood vessels, great for hearts, and fabulous for relationships.

In the last twenty years, children have been taught the difference between good touch and bad touch to empower them to recognize and prevent abuse. We applaud these efforts but believe that the emphasis has been too strong on the avoidance of bad touch—while undermining the positive value of good touch. One example was the story we shared earlier about the middle school that, because of violent incidents, banned all forms of physical contact. Another example comes from John, an after-school-program teacher. He told Larry about a boy who, in the middle of his kindergarten year, came to a new school, eager to make friends. His strategy was to kiss every child who came near. Some of the kids liked this gesture, though most didn't; and the teachers didn't like it at all. John realized the boy needed an alternative way to make friends, so he taught him how to high-five. The boy ran off to immediately try it, shouting, "High five!" and slapping hands with the first kid he saw. It worked!

In other words, when out-of-control violence—or out-of-control affection—is the problem, elimination of all physical contact is *not* the solution. The solution is *more* physical contact, as long as it's positive and mutually enjoyable. Healthy touch is also the antidote to the media's constant emphasis on sex and aggression as the dominant forms of physical contact. Roughhousing sends an alternate message: There are countless healthy ways to be physically close and connected. The world of healthy touch is about friendship, camaraderie, nurturing, and fun—not sex or violence.

Edmund Knighton, a professor at Santa Barbara Graduate Institute, is devoted to bringing good-quality wrestling to children and schools. He advocates wrestling as early as age two or three, as well as throughout childhood, because it's so good for physical and emotional development. However, even when he eloquently explains the benefits for children provided by wrestling—ranging from strength and gracefulness to perseverance and joy—he typically faces resistance from adults worried about the dangers of high-intensity physical contact.

Knighton's best method of overcoming this resistance is one we agree with wholeheartedly: He teaches parents and teachers to wrestle. He starts with standing moves that are cooperative and lighthearted and then guides them through a series of steps (akin to our Warm-Up program in chapter 2; see page 33) until the adults are on the floor really wrestling. "You have to do it yourself to understand that it isn't about violence," he told us. "When children learn how to wrestle this way, they finish with a wonderful sense of exhaustion and a wonderful sense of where they are in their bodies, because wrestling is really a dance and a relationship. It has the appearance of competition, but it is more about tuning in and matching strength than about winning. Wrestling builds relationships, rather than hurting them."

The extreme violence that surrounds us, in real life and in entertainment, can easily lead to confusion about the idea of wrestling. On the surface, high-contact roughhousing and aggression seem to have a lot in common. But look closely at the participants' faces and you'll immediately see the difference. A playful wrestle might look like a fight, but an expression of glee looks nothing like an expression of pain, terror, or rage. Violence creates disruption; roughhousing promotes deeper connection.

Play-fighting is one of life's most social activities, because it's like a dance, with each partner highly attuned to the other. In rats, play-fighting activates the areas of their brains that deal with interactions, sometimes called the social brain, which results in better social skills. Rats who don't wrestle, and rats with injury to the social brain, lose their ability to play or to mate with other rats.

Besides its connection benefits, contact roughhousing also gives children an opportunity to explore their strength and flexibility. This combination is the essence of being an agile person. And we're not just talking about physical agility here, but also mental agility. Athletes are recognized for their physical agility on the playing field. But deep down, they know that they are only as good as their mental agility allows them to be. Anthony Pellegrini points out that play-fighting's short but intense bursts of activity are similar to interval training used by athletes for maximum cardiovascular fitness. All this paves the way for lifelong fitness, instead of screen-induced blobness.

Being in good physical condition raises kids' self-confidence, which helps them face the world waiting for them beyond their homes and neighborhoods. And feeling comfortable in their own bodies is a big help in learning to control their impulses and interact well with peers.

Essential Contact Skills

Practice: For these moves, it is especially important to practice first with a pillow or soft object before "going live" with your child. Practice will prevent a mishap that could turn your flip into a flop. Some of the more challenging flips require a spotter, so make sure your spotter practices, too!

Know Your Limits: Most contact moves require a minimum strength level to safely accomplish them. That doesn't mean you have to be a bodybuilder, but you may need to work on your strength during nonroughhousing hours.

Resistance: You want to provide just the right level of resistance so that your child needs to use a healthy amount of strength to break your hold or take you down. Too much resistance leads to excess frustration and giving up. Inadequate resistance also leads to quitting, because there's not enough challenge. Typically, you start with low resistance and build to higher levels.

Flexibility: Make sure you do a few gentle stretches before attempting the contact moves. Even if you're flexible (and most of us aren't!), some stretching or a yoga class will aid greatly in making the activities more enjoyable for both you and your child.

Self-Handicap: When your child is smaller, weaker, and less confident than you, your job is to handicap yourself, holding back and matching your child's strength. As she grows stronger and more confident, you can turn up the heat. When she gets to the point at which she can take you down, it's her turn to self-handicap!

Just Plain Wrestling

Ages:	2 and up
Difficulty:	Easy
Essential Skills:	Resistance, Self-Handicap

Wrestling is all about rolling up your sleeves, taking off your tie, and getting down on the floor with your kids. On the surface, wrestling appears to be a form of combat, but at its heart it's all about connecting. It's fluid, interactive, and constantly moving. The Japanese word *judo*, the name of the martial art that most closely resembles wrestling, literally translates as "gentle way."

The key to wrestling is to make it a roughly equal match. (That means you hold back when your children are young; as they get older, you step up; and once they can take you, they take a turn at holding back.) If you're taller than your child, start out on your knees or on all fours while he stands. Roll around and grapple together. Take him down, and then allow him to take you down. Stick to pushing, pulling, and rolling. Stay away from lifting, hitting, kicking, body slams, headlocks, or flying elbows. Roughhousing wrestles can be free-form, or they can have specific goals, such as the following:

- Pin the opponent's shoulders to the ground for a predetermined length of time. Make your child really exert herself to keep you down for the count.
- Take turns working to move past each other to reach a finish point on the other side of the room.
- Have your opponent start on all fours while you try to flatten her, either face-up or facedown.
- Push each other out of a specified area, such as a ring on the carpet made from rolled-up sheets or scarves.

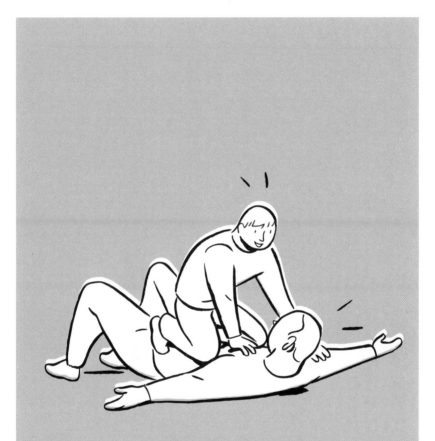

To make it a roughly equal match, hold back with
young children; step it up as they get older.

Crane

Ages:	2 to 5
Difficulty:	Easy
Essential Skill:	Flexibility

This move has its origins in Shaolin Kung Fu and is based on a kick that involves raising one's arms in the air and shift-kicking from one foot to the other. Crane doesn't involve kicking, but the setup is similar to the kung-fu kick.

Stand on a soft surface (carpet, grass, etc.). Invite your child to sit, facing you, on your stronger foot while you hold her hands. Lift your leg in the air and launch her off your foot, holding onto her hands to soften her descent to the ground (*not* onto your foot—plant it firmly back on the ground after the launch). Avoid performing Crane on hard surfaces because, if your child reaches a good height, her landing will hurt.

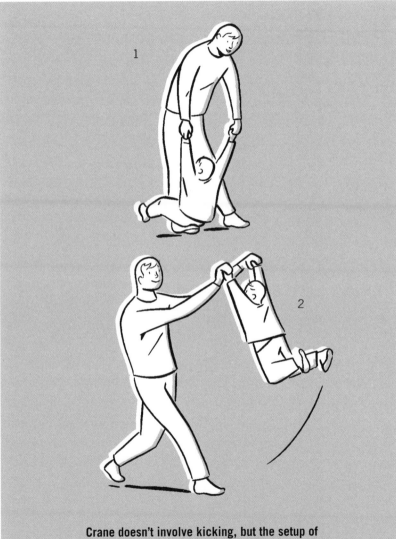

Crane doesn't involve kicking, but the setup of this move is similar to a kung-fu kick.

Steamroller

Ages:	6 months and up
Difficulty:	Easy
Essential Skill:	Flexibility

This move is the epitome of physical contact. Lie on your back and place your child on top of you, belly to belly. Wrap your arms around him. Now roll over together, maintaining belly-to-belly contact, so that he is on his back and you are on top. (Prevent squashing your child by using your elbows to support your weight when you're on top; doing so will also help you maintain a steady speed as you roll.) Continue for three rolls and then reverse, rolling in the opposite direction. Once you master this move on a flat surface, head for a hill.

If your child is less than 18 months old, place one hand on the back of his head throughout the move, and keep almost all your weight on your own elbows.

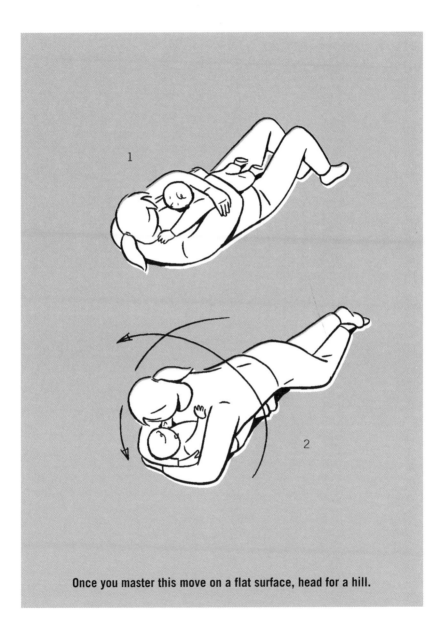

Once you master this move on a flat surface, head for a hill.

Houdini

Ages:	2 to 4
Difficulty:	Medium
Essential Skill:	Know Your Limits

This move, named in honor of the great magician and escape artist, is especially suited for younger children. Imagine that Harry Houdini is tied with heavy chains to a tree and is about to attempt an unbelievable escape. Lie on your back and bend your knees, keeping your legs together and your feet on the floor. Direct your child to sit on your feet; her back should recline onto your shins. Tell her to grab the back of your calves. Now have a sibling, Mom, or a friend wrap a few strands of masking tape (not too tightly) around your child and your calves. Now the daring escape! Lift your legs together off the floor so that your child is now being raised into the air. As she reaches an almost upside-down position, put your hands on her shoulders/chest, shout for her to make her escape (meaning that she rips off the masking tape), and then flip her backward directly over your head.

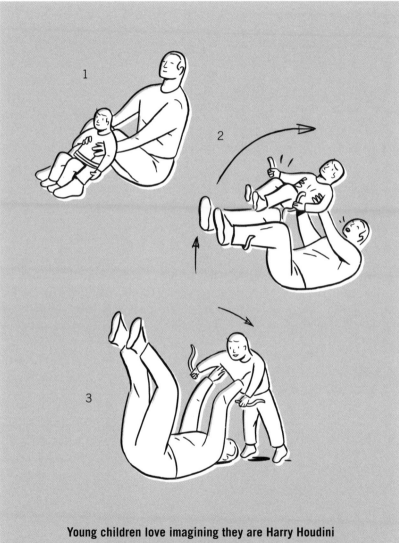

**Young children love imagining they are Harry Houdini
attempting an unbelievable escape.**

K2

Ages:	2 to 7
Difficulty:	Medium
Essential Skill:	Know Your Limits

Nestled between Pakistan's northern territories and Xinjiang, China, is K2—the second-tallest mountain on Earth. In this move, you become a mini-version of K2, and your child attempts a daring ascent! There are three levels: (1) sea level—the ground or mat on which you're performing the move; (2) base camp—halfway up your body, usually hip level; and (3) summit—sitting on your shoulders.

Your child should stand facing you, hold your hands, and start climbing up your legs to the various levels. Once he makes it to the summit, try various dismounts, similar to Empire Bluff (page 120). Base camp is the best spot for him to do a backward flip, with your assistance, back down to sea level.

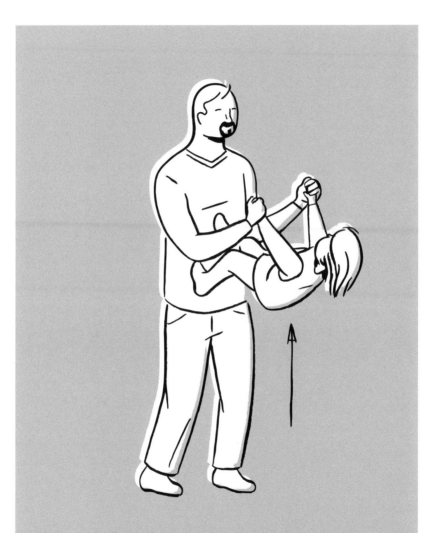

After reaching the mountain's summit, your child can
try various dismounts to return to sea level.

Ninja Warrior

Ages:	Infancy to 2
Difficulty:	Medium
Essential Skill:	Practice

Invite your child to sit on your shoulders. Reach underneath her armpits (inverting your hands so that your thumbs face forward and your fingers wrap around the back of her body). Quickly flip her forward, over your head, off your shoulders, and down to the ground—just as a ninja would somersault off a building—supporting her with your hands the whole way. A great variation for a child two years or older is to allow her to slide down your back on her belly. Start by lifting her off your shoulder via her arms or armpits. Then bend slightly forward and slowly lower her down your back. Once she's about halfway down, you can usually let her slide the rest of the way on her own.

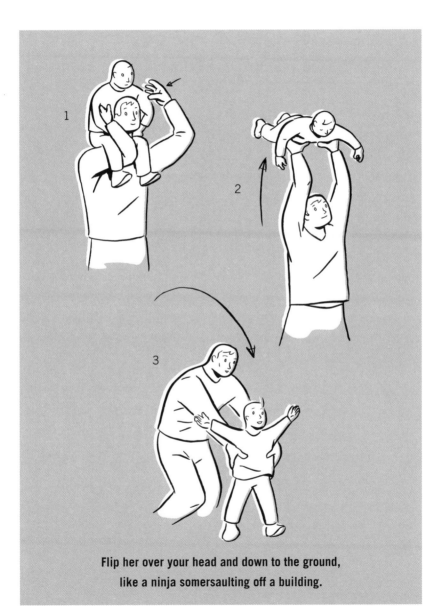

Flip her over your head and down to the ground,
like a ninja somersaulting off a building.

Red Tornado

Ages:	3 to 7
Difficulty:	Medium
Essential Skill:	Practice

Named after the DC Comics superhero whose superpower is the ability to produce high-force winds and extreme forward velocity, this move starts with your child standing with his back to your front, a couple feet in front of you. He then tips his head toward his chest and reaches back between his legs with both hands. Grab his hands or arms and simultaneously lift and flip him over in the air. You're essentially helping him do a somersault in the air, with tornado-force winds! The key is to lift at the same time as you flip; otherwise, you risk cracking his head on the floor. The first few times, a spotter can help with getting his legs up, over, and around. Placing a pillow on the floor under his head is another wise safety precaution.

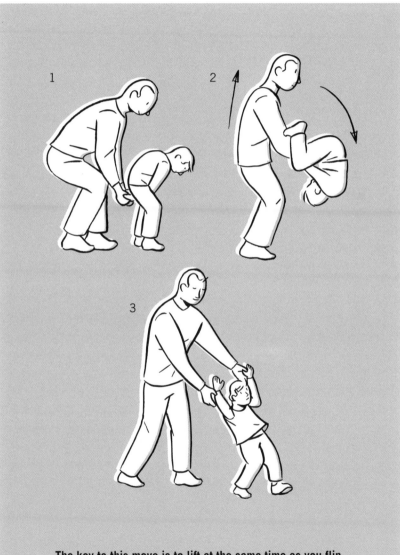

The key to this move is to lift at the same time as you flip.

Yakima!

Ages:	7 to 12
Difficulty:	Medium
Essential Skills:	Practice, Resistance, Self-Handicap

Yakima Canutt is widely regarded as one of Hollywood's greatest stuntmen. Originally trained as an American rodeo rider, Yakima not only taught the craft of performing stunts, he also invented devices to make stunts safer. He often doubled for John Wayne and, in the process, developed a friendship with the Duke. The two, working together, created many of the stunt and screen-fighting techniques still used today.

In this move, you and your child will stage a choreographed fight scene. Below are a few tips and techniques to consider incorporating into your scene. The key is working together and practicing before you do the activity in front of the camera (or Mom!).

TIPS

Minimal contact. Remember, you're not really fighting.

Opponent recoil. This concept is critical for making a play-fight scene believable. The more the person being fake punched and fake kicked recoils in a dramatic, exaggerated way, the better. This includes falling or crashing to the floor.

Follow the child's lead. Does she want to be the outlaw or the marshal?

Rehearse, rehearse, rehearse. The more you practice, the more realistic it will look. Practice your dialogue, too!

TECHNIQUES

Slapping. One performer should do a "slap clap" near his opponent's face for sound effects. Basically that involves slapping your own hand after fake hitting your opponent.

Punching. Hooks are easier to fake than uppercuts or jabs because your opponent can simply recoil his head and body away from the punch (and away from the audience's viewpoint). Either the puncher or the punchee can pound his own chest to simulate the punch's sound.

Kicking. Two styles work well. The first is a mule kick: Turn away from your opponent and kick backward. The second is a knee kick: Grab your opponent's collar and pull him forward into your knee as you lift it (while your opponent does a dramatic whiplash-esque recoil with his head).

Pushing and pulling. Do these moves a lot. When one person falls down, the other should pull him back up for more fun.

VARIATION

Once you've gotten the hang of the techniques, try a slow-motion variation. All the techniques, like punches and recoils, should be done super slowly, including falling and getting back up. In slo-mo, you can have true contact instead of fake contact, and you won't need as much rehearsal, because the safety comes from the slowness of the move.

Empire Bluff

Ages:	2 to 7
Difficulty:	Hard
Essential Skills:	Practice, Know Your Limits

Named in honor of a hiking trail at the Sleeping Bear Dunes National Lakeshore, in northern Michigan, this move involves your child, with your help, doing a forward somersault vertically up your body, ending in a sitting position on one of your shoulders, with his legs dangling down your back. It's one of the more challenging to master, so practice with a pillow or similar prop before going live. Also, if you're left-handed, reverse the instructions below.

Start by standing and facing each other. Direct your child to bend at the waist and put his head between your thighs as if you were going to give him a wrestling pile driver. Grasp his hips and flip him up toward your chest. As you're flipping, use your left leg (which will be against his back as he comes toward your chest) to raise him up. Lift him a little farther until he's sitting on your left shoulder, facing backward, with his legs dangling against your back. At this point, place your left arm and hand around his stomach and position your right hand to support his back. This is known as the Bluff position. From the Bluff, there are multiple dismounts. One is simply pivoting him around on your shoulder (his butt and legs will swing away from your head) and allowing him to slide down your chest to the ground. Another is letting him leap onto a couch or bed behind you. The key to any dismount is to prevent your child from reaching the ground via gravity alone. Break his landing with either your chest, as in the slide technique described above, or your arms or hands (or both).

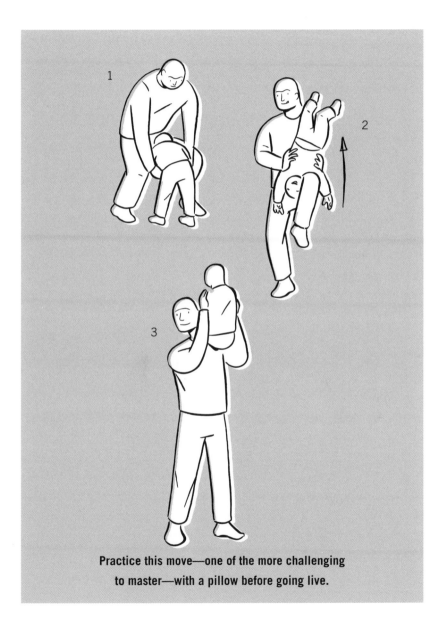

Practice this move—one of the more challenging to master—with a pillow before going live.

Hummingbird

Ages:	12 and up
Difficulty:	Hard
Essential Skill:	Flexibility

The hummingbird is the only bird on Earth capable of flying backward. The male Anna's hummingbird (*Calypte anna*) was also recently named the fastest animal on earth, traveling at speeds in excess of 385 times its body length per second. This move is all about being backward in the air, hence the name. *Note:* You *must* use a spotter. Start by standing back-to-back with your child. Grasp each other's hands (ideally you should be roughly the same height, so shorter children should stand on a chair). Bend forward at the hip and, at the same time, your child should bring his knees to his chest. With one quick motion, stand up and flip him directly over your head and onto the ground. Your hands remain together throughout the entire flip. The spotter's hands should be placed underneath your child's thighs before you begin the flip and guide him throughout the move. An easier version, taken from the swing-dance playbook, is to lock elbows (instead of hands) to do the flip.

Expert variation: Again, this variation *must* include a spotter. Your child stands with his legs apart. Squat behind him and put your head between his legs (so that he is sort of sitting on your neck). Now stand up in one quick motion so that he does a backflip and lands behind you. As you stand, he should bring his knees to his chest. This time, the spotter's hand should be on the child's chest/abdomen to assist with the backflip.

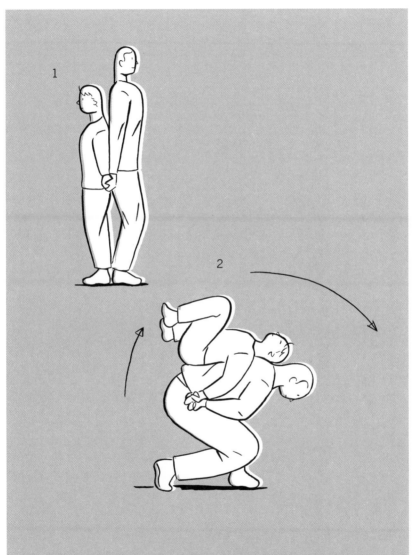

For an easier version of this flip, lock elbows rather than hands.

Pilobolus

Ages:	12 and up
Difficulty:	Hard
Essential Skills:	Flexibility, Know Your Limits

In this move, named after Pilobolus Dance Theater (a troupe known for its athletic prowess), you and your child will perform a series of *connected* forward rolls. Because you will be connected to each other, this move works only with kids who are nearly your height. Start by standing on a mat or soft grass, legs shoulder-width apart. Have your child lie on her back, with her head between your feet. She should lift her legs toward you; you grasp her ankles. At the same time, she reaches back and grabs your ankles. Slowly lower yourself into a forward roll over her legs, bringing her to the standing position to complete the next roll. Repeat.

Important note: Forward rolls may cause dizziness. Try a few by yourself before doing them with your child.

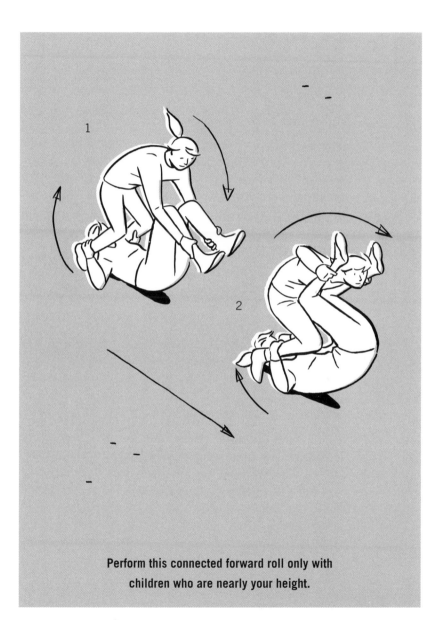

Perform this connected forward roll only with children who are nearly your height.

Real Stories from the Wrestling Mat

At the ripe age of 11, Anthony was into judo, karate, and anything related to ninjas. One day, he decided to test his roundhouse kick on his dad. This story became one of those family legends that is told and retold: *The Incident of the Infamous Buttocks Kick*. It was followed by the longest game of (nonplay) chase the DeBenedet house has ever seen. Once his dad finally caught him, he explained that Anthony was getting older and stronger and that his strength could actually hurt others, including Dad!

When the tide turns and our kids become as strong as we are, or strong enough to hurt us, our job is to teach them to control their strength, just as we did when they were younger. Every family has to figure out an acceptable intensity level for roughhousing. In Anthony's house, that level was pretty high, and acceptable activities included arm-punching contests with his dad. They would take turns tightening their biceps as much as possible and letting the other throw a punch. They traded punches and trash talk ("Dad, I think a fly just landed on my arm and flew away") until someone called it quits with the code phrase, "Wow, that was a good one!" Anthony is pretty sure, looking back, that his dad toned things down for him, but at the time he felt like they were both using their full strength, within the safety of a close father-son relationship. In families that don't play it as close to the edge, this level of play fighting might be too much.

One day, one such family came into Larry's office, hoping he could referee an argument between Mom and Dad. Their son Marcus had been bullied repeatedly on the school playground. Dad thought Marcus should hit back and wanted to coach him on boxing techniques. Mom, not a fan of responding to violence with more violence, wanted Marcus to find more peaceful solutions. In typical therapist fashion, Larry reassured the parents that they were both right. He encouraged them to do lots and lots of rough-and-tumble play at home—no punching, but wrestling and other high-intensity, high-contact moves. Larry explained to Dad that the purpose of this play was to build confidence, not toughness; he encouraged Mom to notice that high intensity is not automatically violent. Marcus listened wide-eyed to this discussion.

Wrestling became this family's favorite activity. Marcus loved when his dad pretended to be a big mean bully—then Marcus would use all his strength to take him down to the floor. This move always ended in a joyful victory lap around the house. Marcus was no longer targeted at the playground, and he never had to throw a return punch. (Most bullies won't target kids who feel physically confident and powerful.) Because he felt more socially confident, Marcus also played more with other, nonbullying kids. After the success of this game, Marcus and his dad adapted it to other challenges and struggles. Dad would pretend to be a hard math problem, a dose of bad-tasting medicine, or any source of frustration, and Marcus would tackle him.

Edmund Knighton, whom we quoted earlier in this chapter, observed that roughhousing contact is especially good for children who are extremely sensitive to certain kinds of touch. They might avoid or feel bothered by specific clothing, sensations, getting messy or dirty, or even being hugged and kissed. Children who have such tactile defensiveness— and it's more common than most people think—are easily overwhelmed by ordinary experiences and therefore miss out on play. Wrestling, strong cuddling, hugging, and step-by-step practice with messy play are simple ways to help these kids become less sensitive and defensive about touch. The key is to tune in to what types of physical contact these children like, what types they can endure, and what types they can't tolerate. Spend lots of time playing with them within their comfort zone and, each day, a little time gently pushing them outside it.

A good example is a five-year-old boy named Levi. He had suddenly become wild, even though his parents tried ensuring that he had adequate sleep, enough exercise, and low sugar intake. None of that made any difference. Neither did time-outs, scolding, or taking away toys. He would randomly walk over to one of his younger sisters and punch her, pull her, grab her, or step on her.

Levi could spend long periods sitting calmly and attentively while his parents read him stories, yet as soon as the story was over he would walk over to someone and pound them. Even his language was filled with violence: "I'm going to break your neck" or "If you say that again, I'm going to cut off your head." That's the point at which Levi's parents asked Larry for help, and at his suggestion they started taking Levi's punches as an invitation for roughhousing play. Now they have all sorts of wrestling matches. Levi's parents challenge him to knock them over or push them off beds, using all his strength but *without* punching or hitting. They have all-out pillow fights; his favorite is when he wears pillows on his arms and legs (putting his hands and feet inside the pillow cases) and knocks his parents over like Sumo-man. His aggression is markedly reduced, and family fun time is markedly increased.

Whenever we ask families for their favorite roughhousing activities, most are variations on wrestling. One mom wrote to us about Earthquake, which she plays with her son:

It started one day when I came home from work and flopped facedown on the bed because I was so tired. My son, who was three, came in and climbed on my back. For a while, he just sat there. I got tired of him sitting on me, so I began to slowly rock back and forth. "What are you doing?" he asked. "It's an earthquake starting!" He giggled. The earthquake got big-

ger and bigger. Finally it got so big that it dumped him off. My son was laughing hysterically, and he climbed right back on for me to do it again. When his sister got old enough, she joined him on my back. They never know when the earthquake is going to hit, and the suspense is nearly as much fun as getting dumped off. When I'm busy and exhausted, I can really tell it affects our kids. They become clingy, whiny, and uncooperative. Twenty minutes of Earthquake restores our connection. And because I can play it while lying down, it's a great game for when I'm really tired.

Here's another story from a parent looking back on how a rough-housing contact game turned things around for a son who was often irritable and depressed. This game demonstrates how pushing—a form of wrestling—is different from hitting or other angry outbursts:

He would get more and more agitated and frustrated over little things and then would blow up. One time, as he was pushing on me in anger, I said, "I bet you can't push me into the other room!" He was already familiar with the wrestling rules, so it only took a couple reminders that hitting and shoving weren't OK. The activity Pushing on Hands was born. We both put out our arms and did basically the opposite of a tug-of-war. Of course, I would gradually let him win, which involved him pushing me into the bedroom and onto the bed, where we would end up giggling. Somehow, this activity would calm his nervous system, like a storm blowing over and the sun coming out. After about three times of me cajoling him into this game, a cool thing happened. Instead of blow-

*ing up, he started to recognize his agitation and would say,
"Mom! I need to push on hands!"*

These stories illustrate the wide opportunities for improvisation in physical contact play. The key to good improvisation is managing the intensity level. You can lower intensity by going in slow motion, by having one child wrestle with you at a time, or by toning down the volume of your voice and reducing your physical strength. You can increase intensity by speeding things up, increasing the volume, and wrestling with multiple kids at once. There is a "sweet spot" for multiple-kid wrestling, in which the older ones aren't too big to hurt you and the younger ones are big enough to get in on the action without getting hurt. Most often, though, one at a time is best, so that each child can go full force. It's difficult to simultaneously intensify the wrestling for one child while lowering it for another!

The other thing to keep in mind when improvising on contact roughhousing is to ensure you're following your child's lead. To illustrate this point, here are two games that seem alike but are in fact very different: One is Tackle, Daddy and the other is Tackle Daddy.

Anthony's friend Dyke and his two-and-a-half-year-old son Avery developed Tackle, Daddy. Every time Dyke returned home from work, his son ran to greet him carrying his football, shouting, "Tackle, Daddy." This was a game they invented together and loved playing. Avery handed the ball to his dad and ran out for a pass (he wasn't yet skilled enough to catch it, but he still loved to try). Dyke threw the ball across the room, and Avery retrieved it. Then Avery ran at his dad at full speed to be tackled. (Apparently, Avery was so excited about the tackling part of the game that he dispensed with the chasing part.) Once they both hit the ground, the game turned to rolling around until Avery said, "Again!" The game would repeat until dinnertime or until Dyke was too tired to continue.

Tackle Daddy was invented by a family who came to see Larry because one of their two daughters was showing serious behavior problems. The dad, Ben, wasn't very involved with his kids, so Larry recommended wrestling as a way for them to form a stronger connection, which he thought might help with their struggles. Ben made it clear that he would "never ever" wrestle with his daughters, partly because they were girls and might get hurt, and partly because he had terrible memories of "wrestling" with his older brother, which was really not wrestling at all but instead involved Ben being beaten up by someone bigger and stronger.

Larry insisted that wrestling could be fun, even for Ben, and that wrestling could be safe, even for his daughters. Eventually, Ben agreed to try it, and together the three of them made up the game of Tackle Daddy. In the game, the two girls would hide in the house, and Ben would walk around looking for them. When he passed their hiding place, pretending not to notice them, they leaped out and tackled him. He screamed for mercy, thrashing his body around vigorously but not using his full strength to throw them off. They never showed him any mercy, of course, except to let him up so they could play the game again. Even though he was pretending to end up helpless on the floor, just as he had been for real with his big brother, Ben was able to experience how different wrestling was when the goal was fun, connection, and empowerment of his daughters.

This game, and the other roughhousing moves the three of them invented after having so much fun, helped the daughter who had been having the greatest difficulties. But, more important, it brought the whole family together. Ben felt, for the first time, like a "real dad," instead of just a breadwinner and disciplinarian. He had learned the power of healthy, playful, physical contact.

CHAPTER 6

Imagination

"In one famous Russian study from the 1950s, children were told to stand still as long as they could—they lasted two minutes. Then a second group was told to pretend they were soldiers on guard who had to stand still at their posts—they lasted eleven minutes."

—Po Bronson and Ashley Merryman in *NurtureShock*

S omething magical happens in the mind of almost every child some-time between the ages of nine and fifteen months: They develop an imagination. Before that age, when you fly your baby around the room, she's just enjoying the movement and the shared excitement. But after that age, she can pretend to be flying, and the activity takes on a whole new dimension. Suddenly a stick can be anything from a bottle to a car. Over time, pretend play becomes increasingly complex and elaborate.

As children reach preschool age, their rapid increase in pretend play promotes social and thinking skills, storytelling talents, creativity, and advanced language. Playing house is a good example. This make-believe activity helps children practice nurturing (just like Mom and Dad), household chores (like Mom and Dad), and arguing (you get the idea). On average, girls are more likely to play house, whereas boys are more likely to engage in good guy/bad guy play acting. But boys need to practice nurturing, too. Otherwise, how will they ever have a clue what to do once they're dads? And how will they learn to solve problems without weapons or super-powers? On the flip side, girls need to explore the emotional territory of anger, assertiveness, and impulse control, instead of just following the "girl rule" of being nice all the time.

Unfortunately, by the time we reach adulthood, the world has brain-washed most of us into thinking we aren't creative. We start believing that creativity is something you're either born with or not. This kind of thinking is dead wrong! Every human being has the full potential to be wildly creative. Some just don't know it's there, or they haven't nurtured it. Also, most people only think of creativity as artistic and musical talent. They're forgetting about the creative power of imaginative play and inspired roughhousing.

It's a good thing that everyone has the capacity for creativity, because creativity is crucial for problem solving. Essentially, if problem solving were a muscle, then imaginative play would be the most effective way to exercise it. Every time children make-believe, they practice the skills required to solve problems. Brian Sutton-Smith, a pioneering play researcher from New Zealand, found that children who were given an unfamiliar object and allowed to play with it were later able to devise more creative uses for it than children who weren't first allowed hands-on play. That is the essence of problem solving—devising multiple solutions. And there's no better way to do this (or learn anything) than by playing. That's why we need more play—not less—both in schools and at home.

The skill of storytelling is often undervalued. Whether the tales are simple or complex, funny or serious, storytelling is crucial in life. It helps us to convey information effectively to others, especially if we want to persuade or motivate them. We love stories that parents tell in collaboration with their kids, bouncing ideas off one another and building something neither one could have thought of alone.

Imaginative play is great. Combined with roughhousing, it's even better. Imagination engages the most creative areas of the mind; roughhousing engages all the muscles in the body; and the interaction between parent and child engages the social brain, which is what gives us the skills we need to get along with other people. The moves in this chapter are especially designed to activate all these areas as you join children in their world of make-believe. In the words of Chris Wink, one of the founders of Blue Man Group and the Blue School in New York City, "Children aren't

IMAGINATION   135

empty boxcars to shovel full of information. We see them as rocket ships; our job is to find the fuse and light it so they can take off."

Essential Imaginative Skills

Divergent Thinking: Also known as thinking of multiple right answers, this process is the essence of creativity. The divergent thinker is endlessly curious, thinks outside the box, knows there is no such thing as a dumb idea, and explores varied solutions instead of settling for one right answer. Props are a great way to stimulate divergent thinking. For instance, a blanket could be a fort or it could be a giant tortilla for a human burrito roll-up. Our favorite props are couch cushions, pillows, mattresses, and blankets.

Role Reversal: Let your child be the strong one, the leader, the capable one, the scary monster, or the savvy hero while you act a little fearful, clumsy, and incompetent.

Storytelling: With all imaginative roughhousing moves, you can add stories, characters, or elements of fantasy. Transforming into various animals is a quick and easy way to get your imagination flowing; experiment with movements, sounds, and emotions. Fantasy superpowers are always a hit, especially if your child has powers you can't compete with. Or pretend to teleport to the extreme edges of our planet. Maybe you'll land on an icy glacier that requires teamwork to rappel down. Or a swamp in the Amazon that you'll need to cross by swinging from vines.

Clifton Bridge

Ages:	3 to 5
Difficulty:	Easy
Essential Skills:	Role Reversal, Storytelling

Spanning seven hundred feet above the Avon Gorge, the Clifton Suspension Bridge is one of the most remarkable structures in the United Kingdom. But will your child dare to cross it alone? Simulate the bridge by sitting on a chair and propping your feet on another; your legs will form the suspension chains. Have your child stand between your legs (like she's a gymnast on parallel bars). Begin swaying your legs. Encourage her to grab "the chains" and hold on tight—it gets windy above the gorge! Use your imagination to invent a host of other perils. Tell her she's come to a hole in the bridge and needs to lift her feet off the ground. Or pretend the bridge has collapsed after being struck by lightning; lower your legs and challenge her to climb up to safety.

You can reverse roles, too. When it's your turn to cross the gorge, keep almost all your weight on the floor but pretend you're wildly off-balance and terrified of plunging into the water. It's a long way down!

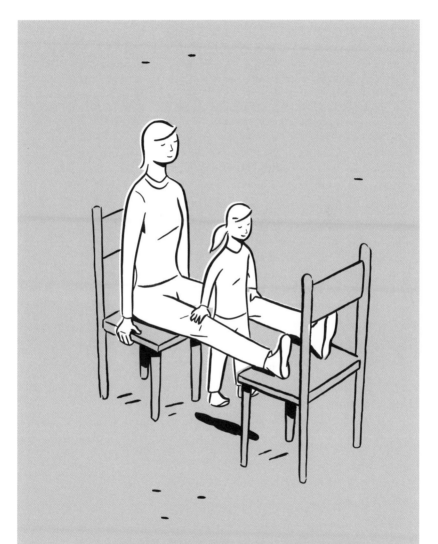

Have your child stand between your legs with her arms over your legs (as if she's on the parallel bars).

Playing (Rough) House

Age:	3 to 6
Difficulty:	Easy
Essential Skill:	Divergent Thinking

This move puts a roughhousing spin on old-fashioned "playing house." It's fine for dramatic play to be calm and quiet, but now and then it's fun to make it a bit more rambunctious.

If your child hosts a pretend tea party, after a few minutes you could jump up and shout, "Oh no! This tea turned me into a dragon, I have to flap my wings," and then start flapping around the room, inviting her to join you. If she puts you in charge of putting the baby doll to bed, pretend the baby is wrestling you wildly and beg your daughter to help you (though she might choose to take the baby's side!). If she announces it's bedtime, say, "I sure hope no one pounces on me while I am sleeping!" Who can resist an invitation like that?

Of course, some children are serious about their tea parties and imagined domestic scenarios, and they do not want you to mess things up by being too rowdy. In that case, go along with their way of playing, *gradually* introducing a few physical elements. Bump elbows as you sip your tea, or say mildly, "Dear me, do I hear a herd of elephants? Should we get all the babies to safety?" If she agrees, you can scoop up the toys—and your child—and jump onto the couch. If she objects, then bide your time and try again later.

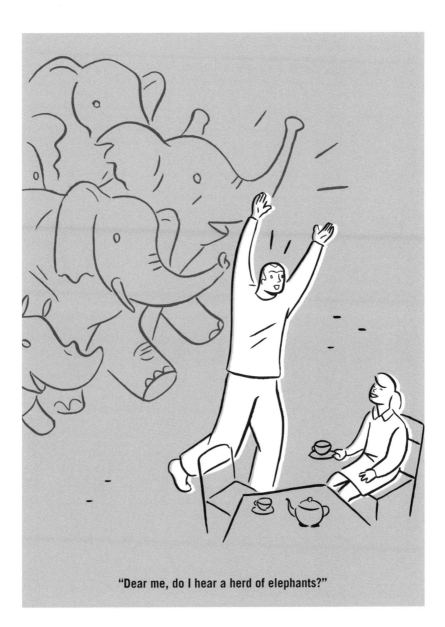

"Dear me, do I hear a herd of elephants?"

The Stick

Ages:	4 to 10
Difficulty:	Easy
Essential Skill:	Divergent Thinking

To the delight of people who love low-tech play, the stick was inducted into the Toy Hall of Fame in 2008. The Strong National Museum of Play, in Rochester, New York, acknowledged the enduring power of the stick as the ultimate creative toy—it can become virtually anything a child wants it to be, instantaneously transforming itself into something new, and it never needs batteries.

To celebrate this honor, we created the Stick, a high-speed imaginative game in which one person chooses an object, hands it to another player, and shouts, "Go!" The person holding the object then calls out as many uses for it as possible, enlisting the other player(s) in acting out the activity. We like to start with sticks and move on to any handy object, from cushions to rocks to mud to raw (or cooked) spaghetti.

Each of the object's uses should flow from the previous action. A stick could start as a shovel digging for pirate treasure, transform into a sword to scare away the pirates, then into a telescope to look for help, next a cane for an old man trying to escape, followed by a key to a hidden cave, and so on. Wild and outlandish activities and acting are encouraged. When the first person runs out of ideas or tires of the task, he or she hands a new object to another player for the next round.

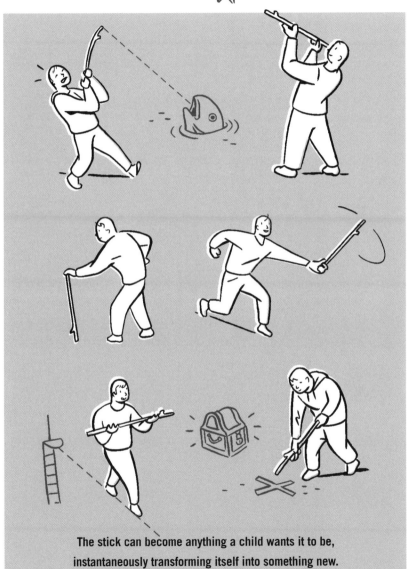

The stick can become anything a child wants it to be,
instantaneously transforming itself into something new.

Alaric the Barbarian

Ages:	3 to 8
Difficulty:	Medium
Essential Skill:	Divergent Thinking

Alaric was the leader of the first tribe of barbarians to capture the city of Rome in 410. In this move, you pretend to be Rome and your child is Alaric. First you'll need to construct Rome. For a fort, use lots of blankets, which you can attach to furniture with masking tape. For a wall, stack up a bunch of sofa cushions. Once you've constructed your ancient fortress, lie down inside and pretend to fall asleep. Your kid will sneak into the fort and land on top of you. Remember to act surprised. Next time, place more pillows or cushions around you, bragging loudly—before you pretend to go to sleep again—that this time your wall will *certainly* keep all barbarians at bay.

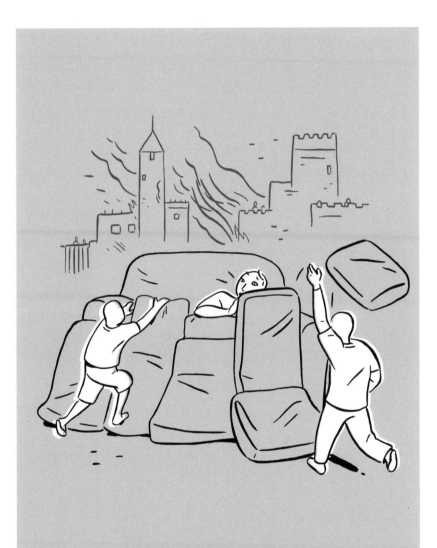

Pillows and sofa cushions are the building blocks of any impregnable fortress.

Big Bad Monster

Ages:	3 to 8
Difficulty:	Medium
Essential Skill:	Divergent Thinking

We learned this imaginative roughhousing activity from a mom whose children invented it with her husband. The idea is this: You sit in a hallway and pretend to be a Big Bad Monster as your children run loops through the house. Each time a child races by, trip them up in some playful way before allowing them to gleefully escape. The monster might hold them in a bear hug, grab their feet, give gentle noogies, or sprawl across the hall blocking the way. Brief obstacles are best so that the kids can run another lap around the house, never knowing what the next go-round will bring but knowing they'll surely be able to break away.

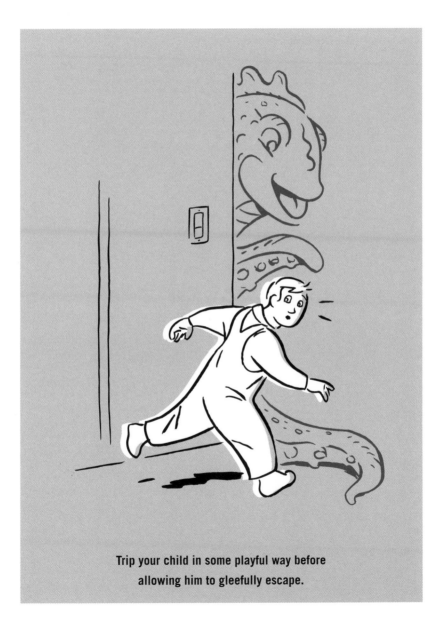

Trip your child in some playful way before
allowing him to gleefully escape.

Magic Carpet Ride

Ages:	2 to 6
Difficulty:	Medium
Essential Skill:	Divergent Thinking

Named after genies' preferred mode of transportation, this move requires a large blanket. It is optimally performed with two or four adults, but can be played solo with a small enough child or a buff-enough grown-up. The child lies down on the blanket and the adults grasp the four corners, take it airborne, and run around. It's an exciting surprise for the child, who can't see what's going on, to bounce the blanket down onto a couch and then lift off again. When only one adult is playing, the child should lie diagonally on the blanket so that his head is pointed toward one corner and his feet toward the diagonally opposite corner; when you lift him, bring together the edges of the blanket like a sack. Lift only 1 to 2 feet off the ground to minimize impact in case of a fall, but beware of grazing the ground as you run. Children often beg to ride in the magic carpet together, but there's too much banging around for it to be safe.

Variation: With at least one adult per corner, and more people on the sides for bigger genies, spread the blanket wide at waist level instead of bunching it into a bundle. Get a rhythm going with little up and down bounces; on the count of three, fling the child into the air. Be sure to catch him a few feet above the ground, so the blanket has room to sag in the middle without allowing him to bang into the floor upon landing. With enough people holding the blanket, your children will love helping to hurl you in the air, if you have the nerve.

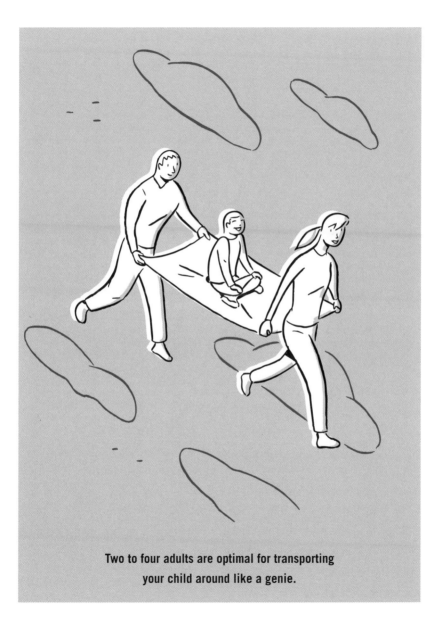

Two to four adults are optimal for transporting
your child around like a genie.

Once Upon a Time . . .

Ages:	3 to 5
Difficulty:	Medium
Essential Skills:	Role Reversal, Storytelling

This activity is designed to combine three things kids love: storytelling, acting out characters, and bashing into people. Decide on a basic topic for your story and turn on appropriate background music (e.g., drums are perfect for an African savannah adventure; electronic music works for an outer-space robot voyage). Begin telling a story that you and your child will act out. Every time you introduce a new person, animal, or creature, everyone becomes that character and acts it out through movements, noises, and lots of physical interaction (like elephant trunks that nuzzle one another, robots that bump into one another, snakes that slither around each other, and so on). Between the appearances of new characters, everyone dances to the rhythm of the music. The story can be silly or serious, invented or based on real life or a movie. Just make sure there are lots of new characters to act out and interact. Try asking kids what should happen next. As your story develops, keep in mind the tried-and-true formula of starting out slow, building up the pace and energy to a crescendo, and then winding down at the end.

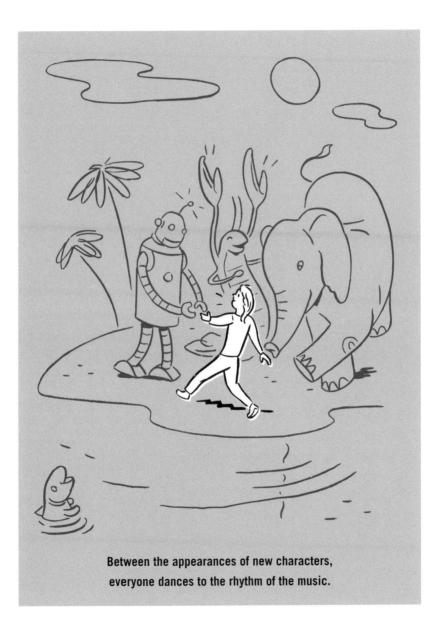

Between the appearances of new characters, everyone dances to the rhythm of the music.

Sasuke!

Ages:	3 to 10
Difficulty:	Medium
Essential Skills:	Divergent Thinking, Role Reversal

Named after the popular Japanese game show in which competitors race through a grueling four-stage obstacle course, Sasuke! is about building your own roughhousing version. Outdoor courses are pretty easy to create. You can use equipment such as cones, nets, balls, and the like, and there's usually a lot of space to set up. Indoor courses are often more challenging because many people aren't sure where to start. Here are a few insider tips.

- **The more furniture you incorporate, the better.** We like big chairs (but not recliners), couches, and sturdy glass-free coffee tables.
- **We also like masking tape, and *lots* of it!** Apply long strips at different heights extending from wall to wall or between pieces of furniture. Pretend they're flesh-eating laser beams that can't be touched. Masking tape works well because it won't pull paint off walls or damage furniture.
- **Pick start and finish points to give your course a direction.** To travel to the finish, jump between pieces of furniture using couch cushions as intermediary landing pads (the floor is molten lava!). Duck under or leap over the masking-tape laser beams, and use teamwork to get through especially difficult laser-beam spots. You can time each other, or just get through it together. Make up stories along the way to explain why you're ducking and dodging.

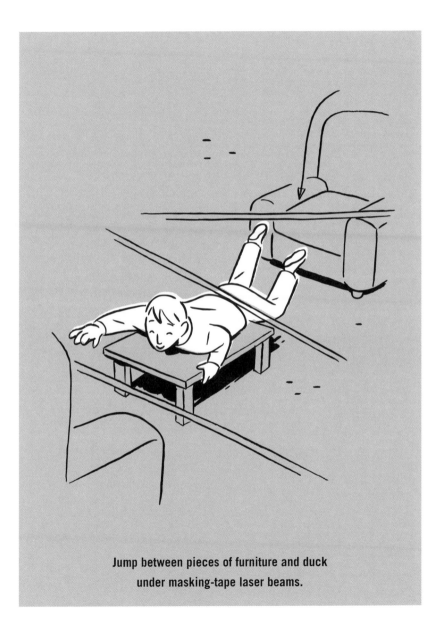

Jump between pieces of furniture and duck
under masking-tape laser beams.

Futaleufú Mattress Rafting

Ages:	3 to 10
Difficulty:	Hard
Essential Skill:	Divergent Thinking

Chile's Futaleufú River is consistently ranked the most dangerous white-water rafting spot in the world. In this move, you'll re-create a trip down the mighty waterway. Grab a toddler mattress, twin mattress, or tumbling mat and place it at the top of a staircase. Jump on the mattress with your child and push off! Hold onto the mattress side handles for stability, but make sure to let go if the mattress is headed for a wall. This move is rated "hard" because of the need for extra caution to prevent crashing into a railing or flipping over on the way down.

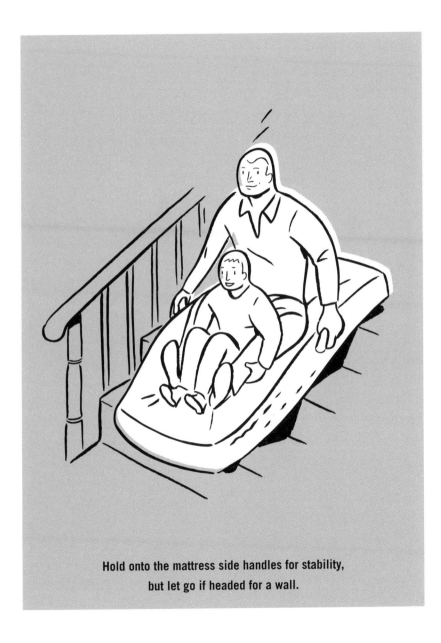

Hold onto the mattress side handles for stability,
but let go if headed for a wall.

Real Stories from the World of Make-Believe

Every type of roughhousing is open to improvisation, but imagination moves *are* improvisation. They're designed to never play out the same way twice, and they provide a great deal of interaction. Even when it's competitive, underneath there's a collaborative dance, and that's a very good thing. As Charles Darwin said, "In the long history of humankind (and animal kind, too) those who learned to collaborate and improvise most effectively have prevailed." Or, in the words of the Grateful Dead, who are of course the *real* authorities on improvising collaboratively: "We abolished the solo in favor of group improv."

Group improvisation means that you and your child work out the details together as you go. For example, one of Larry's clients, a nine-year-old boy named Omar, had never engaged in any fantasy play when he was younger. He was a serious child and had trouble making friends at school. He liked playing chess, so Larry would play—and lose (despite making no effort to do so on purpose). After a few games of silent, serious chess playing, Larry introduced an imaginative element, pretending that he was the wild and impulsive Bobby Fisher while Omar was the stoic Boris Spassky. Whenever Larry lost a piece or a game, he would throw a big fake temper tantrum and chase Omar around the room. The result was that Omar was able to loosen up, engage in more playful play, and make friends with other kids.

Storytelling is a critical skill we can teach our kids through imaginative roughhousing. The combination of movement and meaning is especially powerful. When Anthony's daughter Mia was 18 months old, she and her mom, Anna, attended a dramatic-play class. One of the props used in the class was a giant multicolored parachute. The adults would fly the parachute in the middle of the room and the kids would run underneath it, often crashing into one another. Sometimes the adults would, all at once, throw the parachute up into the air and then quickly pull it behind and underneath themselves, sit down on the edge, and create a parachute fortress with everyone inside. In the middle of the parachute was a small open circle. Mia would always tilt her head upward, gazing through the opening. Together, Mia and her mom made up stories about what was going on up there "in the sky," usually wild stories about dogs flying in the air. Mia loved these stories, which were so different from the stories she liked to listen to at bedtime. The physical aspect of the parachute play sent the creative storytelling off in new, adventurous directions.

As kids grow older, superhero play can become imaginative roughhousing play; all you have to do is add some fun physical contact. Trying to fly is always a good choice; falling flat or crashing into one another is even better. If your child assigns you to be the bad guy, you can play Almost Gotcha (page 35), falling in a tangled heap as your child makes a last-second escape. Most children love to roughhouse right at the edge of where they're scared—but not too scared—so make sure the bad guy or monster you play is a little bit goofy or bumbling. You can boost the scariness with sound effects, increased height, faster speed, and unexpected surprises, but don't overdo it. Watch for any shift from delightedly scared to genuinely frightened. The basic rule of thumb is that children know exactly how much they want to fake scare themselves. When we try to push the fear factor too far or too fast, the result is usually a big upset.

Many children like to play school so they can reverse roles and become the teacher. They often enlist their parents to be students (usually naughty students, because that makes for a much more fun game). There's no reason that your school has to be as controlled and calm as real school.

So why not enroll in Pillow-Fighting School, Dinosaur Battle Conservatory, or the Staircase River-Rafting Academy?

Imagination is a great way to make tired old games, like "horsey ride on Daddy's back," fun again. Instead of just being a horse, you can be a wild stallion racing away from outlaws or a space shuttle heading to Mars. However, some children will have a fit if you try to change any detail of their favorite game. In that case, the best solution is to be extra-enthusiastic, extra-energetic, and extra-exuberant. Doing so shows children that you're willing to play *their* way, which paradoxically inspires them to introduce a little more creativity into their games.

Any roughhousing move is more fun if you act out the parts of silly or extreme characters. When Larry's client Ming plays Alcatraz (page 35) with his son and daughter, they always pretend to be a cruel warden and a pair of dastardly outlaws. Over a few years of playing this game, they developed elaborate voices and personalities for these characters to go along with the physical fun of chasing and capturing. Just when Ming thought the game had run out of steam, his kids added a new twist. Once in jail, they would tell him to stop being the jailer and instead become their getaway horse, leaping onto his back from the sofa-jail.

One day when Ming was especially tired, he made up his own variation. He wanted to play something less strenuous, so he said to them, "Let's play something that won't tire me out so much, but we still get to have fun and cuddle." He suggested something so simple he was sure they would never agree to it: "How about 1-2-3 cuddle?"

"What's that?"

"We count to three, then you two jump into my lap for a giant hug." To his surprise, they loved the idea and played it over and over. After a few times they made it more suspenseful by not telling him what number they were counting to before they leaped onto him.

The combination of imagination and roughhousing has endless variations. A mom wrote to us about her discovery of one that worked for her family, which inspired Booby Trap (page 36):

> *My son and I made up a new game combining resistance and physical connection. He clapped my hands together and then tried to pull them apart. They became magnet hands. He giggled and tried harder to pull them apart. I'd give him just the right amount of resistance before clamping them down again, this time capturing his face between them. His head was stuck in the magnet! My magnets then clamped around his back, over his hands, etc., and each time he just loved trying to break them apart. Also, I keep thinking about how much conflict can be avoided by being silly. Yesterday my husband was putting something in the fridge and my son climbed inside it and said, "Shut the door!" My husband said, "Come on buddy, get out of the fridge." Mark exclaimed, "No!" I could see my husband preparing to argue back. I leaned over to my husband and whispered, "Pretend he's a huge vegetable and you can't shut the door." So my husband said in a loud and silly voice, "Oh my goodness, it's a huge potato! You're the biggest potato I've ever seen! I better shut this door. Ah, no! It won't shut." Mark giggled, then stepped out of the fridge and ran into the other room to play. My husband then turned to me and said, "That is the kind of advice I really appreciate."*

CHAPTER 7

Extreme Roughhousing

"At 211 degrees, water is hot. At 212 degrees, it boils.
And with boiling water comes steam. And with steam, you can
power a locomotive."

—Sam Parker in *212°: The Extra Degree*

We started this book with "Instant Roughhousing," took you through the worlds of "Flight," "Games," "Contact," and "Imagination," and now we conclude with "Extreme Roughhousing." The moves in this chapter are extreme, but so are the benefits: risk taking, perseverance, and confidence.

Risk taking means welcoming challenges, facing them head-on. We don't want our children to blindly ignore potential dangers, but we do want them to be willing to put themselves on the line, to try new things even though they'll probably fail the first time. But it isn't really failure, since success means facing every obstacle, no matter the outcome. This attitude is what the art of roughhousing teaches.

Some children, on the contrary, hesitate to take risks. That's where you come in. Your presence, your close connection with your children, and your confidence all join together to make it possible for them to step out of their comfort zones and right up to the edge. Don't push them over the edge, but don't let them back away, either. These extreme moves are a great place to explore risk taking—just hold their hands and step out into the unknown together.

Perseverance is another great benefit of extreme roughhousing moves. Constant effort, getting back up when you're knocked down—these are the principles behind the quote that opens the chapter: Put that extra 212th degree of effort into everything you do, and you'll be strong enough to power a locomotive!

The tendency for many of today's parents is to make things easy for children. This approach, although well intentioned, prevents them from growing up. Kids need to experience adversity to become adults. They need challenges. Not impossible ones, but significant ones. As Po Bronson and Ashley Merryman write in their book *NurtureShock,* it might seem like the old cliché, "Try, try again," but in fact people who have perseverance "rebound well and can sustain their motivation through long periods of delayed gratification." They describe new neuroscience research about a circuit in the brain that activates in some people—those with perseverance—when things get hard. To develop this circuit, children need some frustration, rather than constant success.

Confidence is also a key to success in life. For every Mozart or Einstein there are many great minds who make no mark, simply because they lack the confidence to send their ideas out into the world. As we've said, many people let their confidence be determined by whether they succeed or fail. But real confidence comes from the mere act of welcoming a challenge or taking a risk, regardless of the outcome.

In addition to risk taking, perseverance, and confidence, extreme roughhousing promotes physical and emotional development. It's obvious that a lot of high-intensity physical play will lower obesity rates. Furthermore, the sustained physicality of roughhousing, punctuated by intense muscle pulses, is the basis for endurance and strength. One long-term study of children documented the relationship between one essential skill of extreme roughhousing—jumping—and bone mineral content. The more jumping a child engages in, the stronger the bones become. And these physiological effects likely persist into adulthood.

The impact of extreme roughhousing on emotional growth is less obvious, but just as powerful. Anthony Pellegrini explains that the way parents and children tune in to one another during vigorous play forms the basis for children to be able to read other people's emotions and signals. Extreme roughhousing is also perfect for children who have a high need for intensity. Does your child slam into you as a way of saying hello? Does he talk loudly, move quickly, and create a tornado of activity? Does he need something to bump up against, always looking for a conflict or a fight? Try out the moves in this chapter and you'll see an immediate difference. When the child's need for high intensity is met through roughhousing, he can settle down and be (a little) less intense the rest of the day.

The moves here are designed to be intense, a little risky, and significantly challenging. If you're a thrill seeker, make sure to keep things safe by tuning in to your child. If risky roughhousing sounds dangerous, remember that real safety comes from knowledge, as Larry discovered when his daughter was three.

One day Emma wanted to stand on the edge of the bathtub with wet feet and walk on it like a balance beam. Larry told her not to, because it wasn't safe. When he turned his back for a second, she climbed onto the edge of the tub. Larry turned around just in time to catch her as she fell. Emma immediately burst into tears. The first thing she said when the crying stopped was, "It was your fault!" Larry explained, not very patiently, that he had warned her it was too slippery.

Emma's response was the essence of three-year-old logic: "You should have known when I was born that I would want to do that." Many years later, Larry and Emma still laugh about that line of reasoning. As outrageous as it was, though, what Emma said bore an element of truth. We should know that our children are born to experiment, to explore, to push the limits.

We can't predict or prevent every disaster, but if we stay alert, we can often be there at the right moment with our hands held out. In other words, if safety comes from knowledge, part of that knowledge is that we can always expect the unexpected from our children. As Emma suggested, they are born to leap into the unknown.

As we grow up, most of us learn to look before we leap. That's fine, but don't forget to leap! Charles Schultz, creator of the "Peanuts" cartoon, once said, "Life is like a ten-speed bicycle. Most of us have gears we never use." The activities that follow will put some of your unused gears into motion.

Essential Extreme Skills

Running: Contrary to popular belief, with practice you can become a faster runner. Teach your child to concentrate on four concepts: knee lifting, forward leg extension, forward arm thrust, and minimal heel strikes.

Jumping: For maximum height, crouch down on your knees and then explode upward, with your arms fully extended vertically. Many people don't realize that a big part of jumping is what your arms do. Add a sprint prior to launch to increase your horizontal jumping ability.

Landing: Landing from heights less than three feet involve simply bending your knees to absorb the impact. For higher altitudes, consult Geronimo! (page 172).

Rolling: The best technique, especially when rolling to disperse impact forces, is a shoulder roll: Bend your knees, lean your head to one side, make ground contact with your hands/arms, and then roll over the shoulder. In the best rolls, your head never touches the ground.

Spanish Steps

Ages:	3 and up
Difficulty:	Easy
Essential Skill:	Landing

Named for the largest and widest staircase in all of Europe, this move is designed to explore the limitless possibilities for extreme roughhousing on stairs. Kids can jump from the highest safe step (never more than six, but start with two or three steps and increase gradually), leaping into your arms or landing on a pile of couch cushions.

Once you've mastered going down stairs, work on going up. Get a running start and see how far up you and your child can jump. Have a contest! Or, with your child sitting on your foot and her arms wrapped around your legs, hop up as many stairs as you can. Once you're at the top, a belly slide back down is always good for a laugh—but you probably don't want to try it unless your stairs are carpeted!

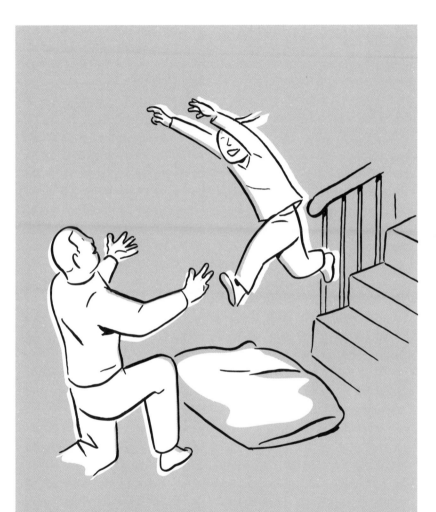

**Kids can start their jumps from the second or third step
and increase gradually to as many as six steps.**

Peter Parker

Ages:	8 and up
Difficulty:	Medium
Essential Skill:	Running

Just as Peter does when he dons his Spiderman outfit, you too can climb walls and help your kids do the same. Stand about 30 feet from a brick wall and sprint toward it from a 30-degree angle (rather than running toward it head-on). The key here is speed, so give yourself a long enough runway to achieve maximum speed. Once at the wall, begin the diagonal climb. You'll likely make it only two or three steps before continuing your run back down and away from the wall. But, with practice, you should be able to reach four steps. When your child makes her attempt, stand at the wall and help her gain altitude by anchoring her at the armpit and hip. Wear tennis shoes with good traction. Another fun variation of Peter Parker is to run at the wall, jump, and plant one foot on it before bouncing off in the opposite direction.

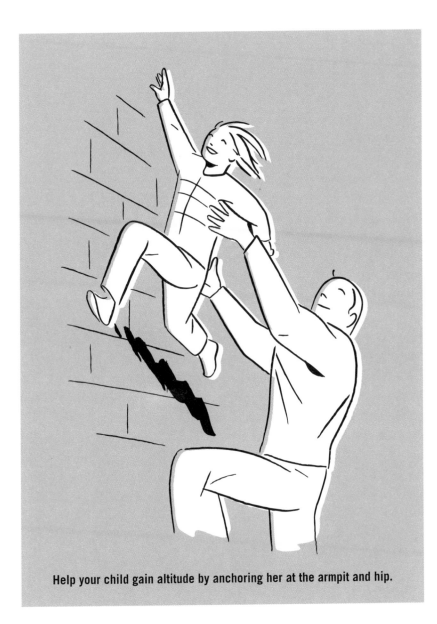

Help your child gain altitude by anchoring her at the armpit and hip.

SEAL

Age:	10 and up
Difficulty:	Medium
Essential Skill:	Rolling

Since their inception in 1962, the U.S. Navy SEALs have been regarded as one of the world's most physically skilled military units. That's due in part to their rigorous selection process, which includes multiple endurance challenges. In this activity, you will create a Navy Seal challenge for your child.

A challenge is a small set of activities (usually two) that the trainee attempts to complete in a certain amount of time. Here's one of our favorites, best done at a lake that has a beach. Position yourself in the middle of the sand, halfway between the water and the grass. Get down on your hands and knees. Slope your back slightly upward from your tailbone to your neck, so that your shoulders are somewhat higher than your hips; maintain contact between the ground and your hands. Have your child lie in an area of grass that's near the sand and several yards away from you. When you say, "Go!" your child should spring up from the grass, sprint toward you, and perform a side roll over your back (so that your backs are touching during the roll). The key for the child is to drop his leading shoulder while tucking his leading arm across his chest. After the roll, have him continue sprinting down the beach and into the water. Have him swim out a certain distance and then head back to shore for another roll over you. The challenge ends when he is belly down again in the grass, right where he started.

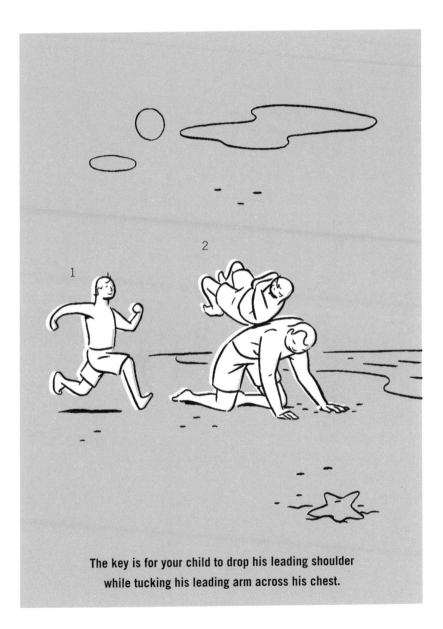

The key is for your child to drop his leading shoulder
while tucking his leading arm across his chest.

Cat Leap

Age:	10 and up
Difficulty:	Hard
Essential Skill:	Jumping

Parkour is the practice of training to overcome physical obstacles, such as buildings, by adapting one's movements to the environment. Cat Leap is a technique used by Parkour artists for jumping onto and over walls.

Choose an outdoor wall whose top is within a "jump's reach" for your child (the height will vary depending on your child, but the jump reach is probably 24 to 36 inches taller than his height). Tell your child to sprint directly toward the wall. When he's a few feet away, have him start his jump, instructing him to jump both vertically and horizontally. He should plant his feet on the side of the wall while grabbing the top with his hands. Then he should immediately use his momentum, as well as his hands and feet, to hoist himself up onto the wall.

There is a natural instinct to come all the way to the wall before jumping, but the problem is there is also an (even stronger) instinct to slow down as you get close; help your child overcome these instincts, since speed and momentum are crucial elements of this move. You should stand at the wall as a spotter until your child gets the hang of it. Challenge yourself by finding a higher wall for you to leap over!

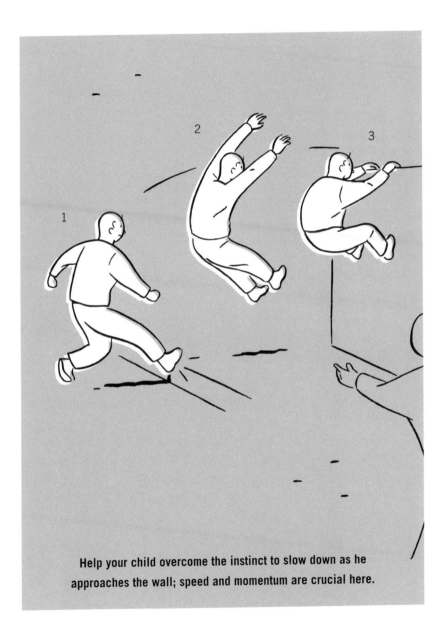

Help your child overcome the instinct to slow down as he approaches the wall; speed and momentum are crucial here.

Geronimo!

Ages:	12 and up
Difficulty:	Hard
Essential Skill:	Landing

World War II paratrooper Aubrey Eberhardt was the first to scream the name of this Chiricahua Apache military leader while jumping out of airplanes. He believed that doing so would free his soul from fear. He probably didn't know that the literal translation of Geronimo is "one who yawns."

In this move, you and your child (twelve years and up only) jump off a deck or roof not more than 10 feet high; garage roofs work well. Here are the basics of high-altitude landings.

- Keep your feet and legs somewhat together so that they hit the ground simultaneously.
- Bend your knees on impact to absorb the impact. (With straight legs, impact forces can be up to thirty-six times greater.)
- Perform an immediate shoulder roll on impact to disperse the forces across a greater surface area.
- Take turns jumping with your child; jumping separately will prevent you from interfering with the other's rolls as you land.
- Climb on top of garages via a tree, ladder, or nearby (and slightly higher) house window. Don't even think about the gutter method.
- Practice jumping from lower perches before trying the real thing!

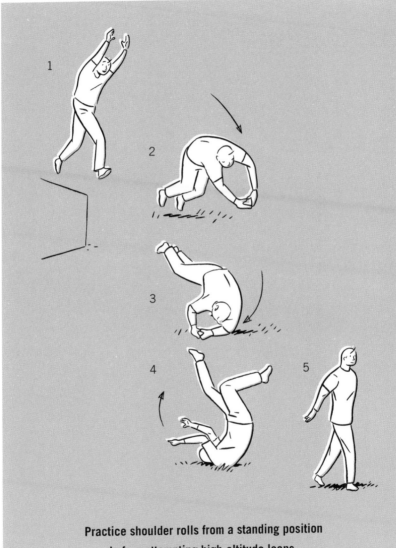

**Practice shoulder rolls from a standing position
before attempting high-altitude leaps.**

It Don't Mean a Thing

Ages:	10 and up
Difficulty:	Hard
Essential Skill:	Landing

As Ella Fitzgerald sang, "It don't mean a thing, if it ain't got that swing." In this move, you and your child attempt a challenging swing-dancing lift. Feel free to turn on a little upbeat music for this one. (If you have swing music, even better.) Also, use a spotter until you're comfortable with the move, especially for the flip.

Tell your child to run toward you; a few feet before she reaches your legs, she should go into a handstand position. As she's in the handstand, reach out and grasp her at the waist, flipping her upward and toward you. As her legs approach your shoulders, you should release her into the air. She should spread her legs (so that she clears your shoulders) as she's descending. Have her wrap her arms around your neck as she comes down; meanwhile, grab her waist to guide her down and soften her landing.

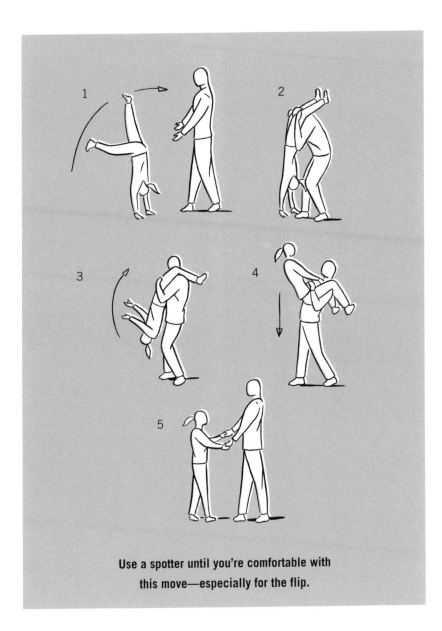

Use a spotter until you're comfortable with this move—especially for the flip.

Vault

Ages:	12 and up
Difficulty:	Hard
Essential Skill:	Jumping

In this move, you explore vaulting via a technique known as "side-planting." Run toward an object from its side, such as the bench side of a picnic table, and plant your palms on it. Then twist your body and lift your legs up and over the object, essentially swinging them around to the other side. In this approach, the front of your chest will be facing the object as you soar over it. When your child is first learning this move, you should spot her on the landing side of the object. Side-planting can also be done with one-handed plants (using the leading hand), but this move requires significantly more strength and agility.

The super-extreme version involves approaching the object head-on. This technique, adopted from the world of Parkour (see Cat Leap, page 170), can be used to leap over most objects that are about waist high. Run toward a low wall or barrier. Plant your hands straight out in front of you so that they hit the wall before the rest of you; they should be slightly wider than shoulder width. Tuck in your legs, bringing them forward through your hands as you jump over the wall. Use your hands and arms as springs to help propel you over the object, landing on the opposite side.

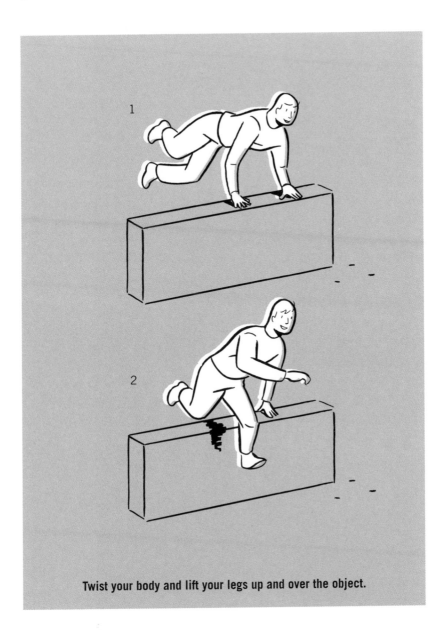

Twist your body and lift your legs up and over the object.

Underdog

Ages:	7 to 10
Difficulty:	Hard
Essential Skills:	Running, Landing

One of the greatest things as a child is to get an "underdog" from an adult while on a swing set. This move is the extreme version—because there's no swing set!

Underdog requires a spotter and a mattress. It's best performed outside, so make sure to grab an old mattress that can get dirty (we like to have a specially designated "outside" mattress). Stand at the edge of the long end of the mattress (but not *on* it), facing away from it. Tell your child to sprint toward you. When she's about 5 feet away, she should put her hands on the ground and do a front handspring directly into you. You will then place your hands under her butt and back and then, with the spotter's help, lift her up and launch her over your head. She should land on her feet on the mattress and then roll forward to disperse the force of impact.

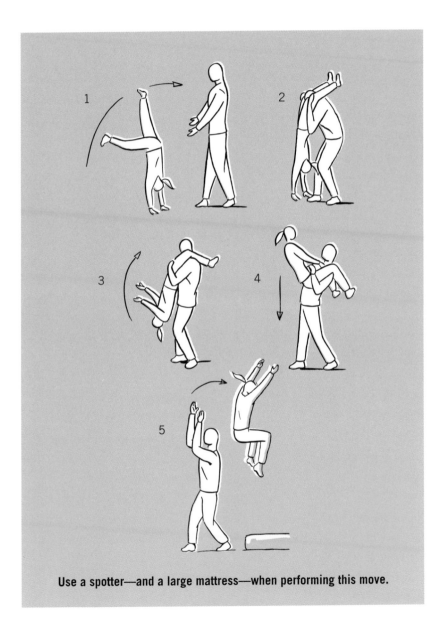

Use a spotter—and a large mattress—when performing this move.

Real Stories from the Edge

Leo was a fearful boy who had a hard time in his kindergarten classroom. He was, according to his parents, always polite to adults and kind to his younger sister. They brought him to see Larry, and Leo was eager to learn techniques to reduce anxiety, which helped somewhat. But the big breakthrough came when Larry visited Leo at home. At first, Leo's play was calm, quiet, highly organized, and careful. Larry didn't let *that* go on for too long! He started increasing the energy level, making Leo's play a little rowdier. First, Larry knocked the engines off the carefully constructed railroad track. Then, he kept bumping his train into Leo's train. Soon, Leo and Larry were racing around the playroom, shouting and laughing. When Leo started hurling trains and screaming at his sister, Larry intervened to tone things down.

Leo's parents were shocked. They had never seen this side of Leo (or Larry!). Like many anxious children, their son worried that, if he ever got angry, he would be horribly violent and destructive. But once he was encouraged to be a little wild and show that he had aggressive impulses just like every other child, he could let go of his fears. Even his younger sister enjoyed the benefits of this change (though he sometimes started teasing her and grabbing her stuff). She loved high-impact play and now could convince him to join her in the physical fun. His parents had a hard time believing that this rowdiness had been inside their sweet little boy all along, but they saw the benefits, too. While watching the two kids running wildly around the basement playroom, Leo's dad said to Larry, with a sigh: "To paraphrase the old song, I guess I have to learn to 'Love the Son You're With.'"

Like Leo, Penny was a cautious child. She always colored inside the lines, never took chances, didn't like to get dirty, and refused all invitations to rambunctious play. Her dad, George, was worried that she would miss out on tons of fun in her life if she didn't get over these inhibitions, so he tried coaxing her, pushing her, teasing her, yelling at her, and begging her. Not surprisingly, none of that worked.

Not one to give up easily, George was always trying new approaches, and one day he stumbled on success. Penny was sitting on the couch reading, and George said to her, "Oh no, be careful, you might fall off the couch!" She giggled. He was making extra-sure that she didn't feel like he was making fun of her, because she was so sensitive. But he had a big smile on his face, and Penny knew he was playing, so she didn't get upset.

She got off the couch, and George followed her, saying, "Oh no, you're not going to *walk*, are you? I can't watch!" He put his hands over his eyes and dramatically bumped into things as he tried to pretend not to look at her in case she fell. She began to do slightly more daring things, to get her dad to pretend to freak out. George played his part perfectly, keeping it funny by pretending he was terrified of her doing "dangerous" things, like walking up and down the stairs. Soon she was leaping off the stairs into his arms and walking along the back edge of the couch. Meanwhile, they both laughed a lot. Once or twice, as Penny increased her daring behaviors, she slipped, and George was right there to catch her, which reinforced that it was OK for her to take these risks. George was surprised to see that Penny's risk-taking behavior extended beyond physical hazards; her drawing, writing, and social interactions became bolder as well.

After playing this way a few times, George called Anthony for some tips on more extreme roughhousing. Once Anthony found out that Penny was especially proud to have overcome a fear of jumping, he suggested several activities for her to try. Her favorite was Peter Parker (page 166), which she performed on the wall outside her school.

While Leo and Penny were cautious children, our friend Jerome was a cautious dad. Jerome's son Daniel, however, was not a cautious child. He loved adventure, and Jerome was constantly exhorting him to "be careful!" One day while at the park, Jerome was hovering nervously near his son, as usual. A nearby mom said, "He looks pretty steady up there. He's a really strong climber." Jerome was about to dismiss her comment as lunatic ravings—how could anyone feel steady when they were climbing so high?—but he looked at his son with new eyes and saw that, indeed, Daniel was very steady. He swallowed his worry and asked Daniel if he was ready to climb higher. Daniel shouted, "Yes!" Jerome asked if he should come up and help. Daniel shouted, "No!"

Today they are both avid rock climbers. Once Jerome embraced Daniel's extreme style, he realized that he might like to try something that had always scared him. So he started rock climbing and introduced Daniel to the sport as soon as he could. They have way more fun together getting wild and rowdy than Jerome ever thought possible.

It's too bad they don't live near an adventure playground. Chances are you don't live near one, either, because they aren't nearly as common as they should be. Adventure playgrounds originated in the 1940s, when a Danish landscape architect noticed that children preferred playing with discarded lumber and piles of rubble to climbing on his carefully designed playground equipment. Though the adventure-playground trend caught on in Europe, only a few exist in the United States. At these amazing play places, kids can build forts and tree houses, make fires in fire pits, and generally do all the things they're usually told not to do. That kind of play is very much in line with the principles behind extreme roughhousing.

Mario wasn't thinking about risk taking when he came to see Larry for help with being a stepparent. He was upset that the close relationship he had built with his stepson Rudy seemed to be on the rocks. Mario could no longer relate to Rudy, couldn't pull him away from his video games or his computer. Instead of horsing around, as they had done when first getting to know each other, now they either argued or kept their distance from one another. To Mario's credit, he was unhappy with this situation, knew it wasn't all Rudy's fault, and wanted to do something about it.

Larry suggested brainstorming things they both might like to do, now that Rudy was a little older. Mario couldn't think of anything and vetoed all Larry's suggestions, saying, "Nah, he'd never go for that." He left Larry's office pretty discouraged, and Larry didn't expect to hear from him again. A few days later, though, Mario sent Larry an e-mail saying that, on his way home, he had a "brilliant idea." He asked Rudy, "How would you like to learn to land safely so that you can jump off the garage roof?" Rudy's mom came home to see Rudy shout at the top of his lungs and jump off the garage, make a perfect roll landing, hug his stepdad, and then shimmy up the tree to the roof again. If it hadn't been for that hug, she said, she would have started screaming.

A few months later, Mario sent a follow-up note. Besides being closer with Rudy and having more adventures together, the roof jumping had an unexpected side benefit. Rudy had always been someone who gave up easily if something was hard. But the idea of this leap was so exciting that he was willing to practice landing for a long time before heading up to the roof, and the idea of getting really good at it was a motivation for him to continue to practice. That's why we include perseverance as a core benefit of extreme roughhousing.

We all know that if we tell highly active children "No" all day long, they're only going to be frustrated and resentful, and so are we. The alternative is to play with them in ways that use their strengths—high intensity, high energy, and fearlessness—and require skill, practice, and focus. In other words, extreme roughhousing. Keep in mind that playing *together* is a crucial part of this formula. If Mario had said to his stepson, "Why don't you go outside and jump off the roof," Rudy probably wouldn't have learned much about landing safely. And Mario would have landed in hot water with Rudy's mom. But doing it together made it a completely different experience.

Some children, though not exactly hyperactive, have an extremely high need for intensity. These kids greet people by hitting or body slamming them; they tend to talk loudly, move quickly, bump into things, and react dramatically to the word *no*. They're often misdiagnosed as having ADHD, but what they really need is more high-intensity play. Wild pillow fights are good, especially with really big pillows safe for fun body slamming. These children often like to be wrapped up in blankets—there seems to be something soothing about being firmly swaddled—and either rolled or carried around the house. Vault (page 176) and Underdog (page 178) are great for high-intensity kids because of the high-speed impact involved. Some parents worry about encouraging high-impact play, but since these kids are guaranteed to do similar stunts on their own, you might as well embrace it, be part of it, and help them do it safely.

A great way to promote perseverance and confidence in children— and ourselves—is something we call Challenge Time. Think of something that would be a physical challenge for your child, maybe climbing a tree, taking off training wheels, or jumping across a small stream. Challenge your child to do it while you cheer her on, providing positive encouragement and support, as described in SEAL (page 168). Then, since fair is fair, let *her* set up a challenge for *you*. (What kind of challenge? We bet there's at least one extreme move that you skipped over.) Go ahead, try it!

The Joy of Roughhousing

"I don't think it is too much to say that play can save your life. It certainly has salvaged mine. Life without play is a grinding, mechanical existence organized around doing the things necessary for survival. Play is the stick that stirs the drink. It is the basis of all art, games, books, sports, movies, fashion, fun, and wonder—in short, the basis of what we think of as civilization. Play is the vital essence of life. It is what makes life lively."

—Stuart Brown in *Play*

T he art of roughhousing is the art of physical, interactive, rowdy play. You know you're in the zone when your child's energy level goes up, his physical activity increases, and exuberance bursts forth. This kind of wild play is totally different from hyperactivity or aggression. You can tell by the joy and sparkle in the child's eyes, the freshness and vitality of the playing, and his desire for more playful physical contact with you. After some high-quality roughhousing, children are happy, content, and seeking closeness. They might even be more cooperative!

When you roughhouse, you send a message to your children that you want this deep connection as much as they do. You also convey that you want them to be safe and adventurous, competitive and cooperative, strong and tender.

If you played your way through this book, you and your children developed courage, confidence, and trust in one another while doing flight moves, launching them in the air and catching them safely in your arms. You fostered teamwork and a healthy competitive edge through roughhousing games, and you increased agility and connection through contact moves. You powered your child's imagination, fueling creativity, problem-solving skills, and storytelling talents. You learned how to be safe through knowledge, supervision, and practice, instead of through rules and saying *no*. Finally, you took everything to the edge in extreme roughhousing, developing perseverance, risk taking, and confidence.

But forget all that.

The real benefits of roughhousing are joy and love. We talked a little about joy in the beginning of this book, and we'll end here with love. There is nothing in the world like active physical play between a parent and a child to bring out deep feelings of love and affection. When you explore and build on these feelings when your kids are young, you set yourself up for a meaningful relationship with them when they become adults. This is especially true for many dads who did not have much practice with nurturing when they were growing up. From the very first time you get a smile from your baby by swinging her gently in the air to working together on challenging roughhousing moves, you and your child will find a deepened sense of close, warm, loving connection.

And that is what it's all about.

Notes

Chapter 1
For more on the play-fighting of ants, see Brown, 2009 (citing ant expert E. O. Wilson, p. 29). Coordinated activation is discussed in Cozolino, 2002; parental contributions to language development are discussed in Fein and Fryer, 1995; the Connecticut middle-school case is documented in the CBS broadcast.

Chapter 5
The social brain is discussed in Pellis and Pellis, 2007.

Chapter 7
See Pellegrini, 2009, for the study on jumping and bone mineral content.

References

Bekoff, M. (Ed.) (2004). *The Encyclopedia of Animal Behavior*. London: Greenwood Press.

Bekoff, M., & Pierce, J. (2009). *Wild Justice: The Moral Lives of Animals*. Chicago: University of Chicago Press.

Bronson, P., & Merryman, A. (2009). *NurtureShock*. New York: Hachette.

Brown, S., with Vaughn, C. (2009). *Play: How It Shapes the Brain, Opens the Imagination, and Invigorates the Soul*. New York: Penguin.

Carson, J., Burks, V., & Parke, R. (1993). Parent–Child Physical Play: Determinants and Consequences. In K. Macdonald (Ed.), *Parent–Child Play: Descriptions and Implications* (pp. 197–216). Albany: State University of New York Press.

CBS Broadcasting, Inc. (2009). Connecticut School Bans Physical Contact. Retrieved April 26, 2010, from http://wcbstv.com/local /school.bans.hugs.2.969949.html.

Cohen, L. (2001). *Playful Parenting*. New York: Ballentine Books.

Cozolino, L. (2002). *The Neuroscience of Psychotherapy: Building and Rebuilding the Human Brain*. New York: W. W. Norton.

The Dalai Lama (1991). *Freedom in Exile: The Autobiography of the Dalai Lama*. New York: Harper Collins.

Des Georges, S. (2009). "ASU to study power of affectionate physical contact." *Arizona State University News*. Retrieved April 26, 2010, from http://asunews.asu.edu/20090205_affectionstudy.

Fein, G., & Fryer, M. (1995). Maternal Contributions to Early Symbolic Play Competence. *Developmental Review*, 15, 367–381.

Fry, D. (2004). Rough-and-Tumble Play in Humans. In A. Pellegrini & P. Smith (Eds.), *The Nature of Play: Great Apes and Humans* (pp. 54–88). New York: Guilford Press.

Goleman, D. (1995). *Emotional Intelligence: Why it can matter more than IQ*. New York: Bantam Doubleday Dell Publishing Group, Inc.

Harlow, H. (1962). The Heterosexual Affection System in Monkeys. *American Psychologist*, 17, 1–9.

Panksepp, J. (2004). *Affective Neuroscience: The Foundations of Human and Animal Emotions*. New York: Oxford University Press.

Parker, S. (2005). *212°: The Extra Degree*. Dallas: Walk the Talk Co.

Pellegrini, A. (2009). *The Role of Play in Human Development*. Oxford: Oxford University Press.

Pellegrini, A. (2005). *Recess: Its Role in Education and Development*. New Jersey: Lawrence Erlbaum Assoc.

Pellegrini, A. (1995). In A. Pellegrini (Ed.), *The Future of Play Theory: A Multidisciplinary Inquiry into the Contributions of Brian*

Sutton-Smith (pp. 194–199). New York: State University of New York Press.

Pellegrini, A. (1991). Children's Rough-and-Tumble Play: Issues in Categorization and Function. In L. Weis, P. Altbach, G. Kelly, & H. Petrie (Eds.), *Critical Perspectives on Early Childhood Education* (pp. 139–152). New York: State University of New York Press.

Pellis, S., & V. Pellis. (2007). Rough-and-Tumble Play and the Development of the Social Brain. *Current Directions in Psychological Science,* 16(2), 95–98.

Reed & Brown. (2005). In K Burriss & B. Boyd (Eds.), *Outdoor Learning and Play Ages 8–12* (pp. 77–84). Maryland: Association for Childhood Education International.

Smith, P. (2010). *Children and Play.* Hoboken, NJ: Wiley-Blackwell.

Sunderland, M. (2006). *The Science of Parenting.* New York: Dorling Kindersley.

Sutton-Smith, B. (2001). *The Ambiguity of Play.* Cambridge: Harvard University Press.

Wipfler, P. (2010). *The Vigorous Snuggle.* Retrieved April 26, 2010 from http://www.handinhandparenting.org/csArticles/articles/000005/000535.htm.

Index of Activities

Acknowledgments

The following people have given life to this book in unique ways: Anna DeBenedet, Liz Wollheim, Ava DeBenedet, Emma Cohen, Mia DeBenedet, Jake Wollheim-Hatch, Lola DeBenedet, Karen DeBenedet, Nelson DeBenedet, Patty Wipfler, David Fuelling, Joe Kimble, MaryAnn Pierce, Millie DeBenedet, Marjorie Kimble, Aaron Timm, Sandie Timm, Nathan Timm, Kim Daly, Lowell Timm, Kathi Timm, Cory Wernimont, Dyke McEwen, Ryan Zaklin, Jacob Towery, Michael McNamara, John Del Valle, and Jason MacIver. Thank you all.

We especially thank Amy Nielander for her energy and creativity, which provided us with an initial spark. We're also grateful to Carl Wiens (for his rowdy illustrations), Doogie Horner (for his rough-and-tumble design), and Mary Ellen Wilson (for her full-contact copyediting). Finally, we are indebted to Jason Rekulak, for making it all possible.

Come play with us online at theartofroughhousing.com.